T0179706

Anatomy of the Heart by Multislice
Computed Tomography

Anatomy of the Heart by Multislice Computed Tomography

Francesco Fulvio Faletra, MD

Head of Cardiac Imaging Laboratory
Fondazione Cardiocentro Ticino
Lugano, Switzerland

Natesa G. Pandian, MD

Professor of Medicine
Co-Director, Center for Cardiovascular Imaging
Tufts University Medical Center
Boston, MA, USA

Siew Yen Ho, PhD

Head of Cardiac Morphology
National Heart and Lung Institute
Imperial College London
London, UK

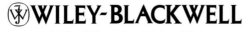

A John Wiley & Sons, Ltd., Publication

Contents

A CD-Rom with video clips is included at the back of the book.

Preface

Anatomy is perhaps the simplest of medical sciences, requiring little more than some curiosity plus careful observation of things as they are.

The new multislice computed tomography (MSCT) machines produce a volume data set with the highest isotropic spatial resolution ever seen. The 0.6-mm "pixel" (picture element) that CT has traditionally delivered in axial planes (x and y dimensions) is also extended to the z dimension as well. The spatial resolution of these new machines is such that they can scan a 10-mm diameter piece of heart in 20 axial sections to produce nearly 4000 pixels for each slice. In other words, these scanners are capable of digitizing the anatomy of a 70-kg human body into over half a billion individual voxels (volume elements).

Given this high spatial resolution, MSCT offers superb 3D images of the entire heart and great vessels. Relationships between cardiac structures can be shown as never before. Electronic casts and electronic dissections of the heart in any plane can show the internal and external cardiac structures.

As a result, the anatomy of the heart and great vessels can be understood easily by young doctors, medical students and nurses. This atlas has been made for them.

MSCT is unique in its ability to image coronary arteries and it is likely to become one of the most used cardiac imaging techniques. Images of coronary vessels provided by MSCT can be interpreted both from radiological and cardiological standpoints. Indeed, radiologists are often not sufficiently familiar with cardiac anatomy, whereas cardiologists often lack adequate familiarity with the axial, coronal or sagittal planes used for visualization of cardiac MSCT images. This atlas has also been made to clarify the anatomy for both specialties.

The atlas is divided into 10 chapters. In each chapter, the body planes, cardiac planes and cardiac structures, such as cardiac chambers, cardiac valves, septa, coronary arteries and coronary veins, are displayed from many perspectives to give the reader a wider vision of living cardiac anatomy.

Acknowledgments

We wish to express our gratitude to Tiziano Mocetti, Elena Pasotti and Angelo Auricchio. This book would not have been possible without their support. We also appreciate and thank Chiara Carraro and Ermidio Rezzonico, technicians at the Radiology Department of Ospedale Civico in Lugano, for their skilful work.

Natesa wishes to thank his students and colleagues from whom he has learnt a great deal.

Ho wishes to thank the Cardiac Morphology team at the Royal Brompton Hospital for their continuing support.

Francesco Fulvio Faletra
Natesa G. Pandian
Siew Yen Ho

Video clips on CD-ROM

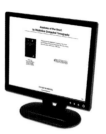

A companion CD-ROM with video clips is included at the back of the book

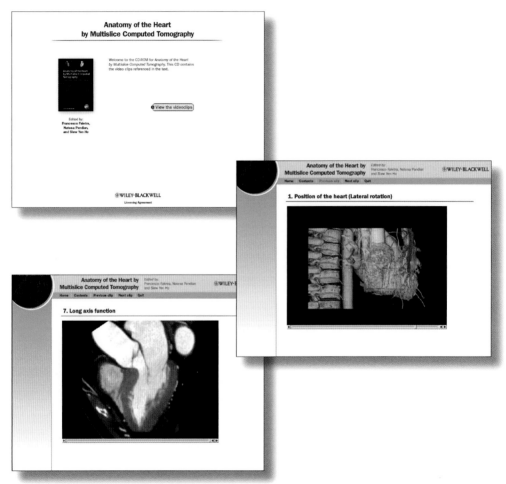

All video clips are referenced in the text where you see this symbol.

CHAPTER 1

Basic Principles

The images of this atlas are derived by a multislice computed tomography (MSCT) machine using the post-processing algorithms available. A brief, basic description of how the machine works and how the algorithms produce different image modalities is given in this introductory section. For more comprehensive descriptions of the post-processing algorithms see "Suggested reading".

The machine

The CT scanner has a ring with an x-ray tube on one side and detectors on the opposite side. This tube-detector unit rotates around the patient during data acquisition. The information (x-ray attenuation) obtained from the detectors during this rotation is processed through a computer, which can calculate the exact attenuation of a given point (pixel) in the examined volume. The width and length of a pixel depend on the size of the detector. With modern spiral CT (Fig. 1.1), the table moves through the ring so that the machine acquires data in a spiral trajectory during tube-detector unit rotation. This makes it possible to acquire attenuation information for a given point in a volume (three-dimensional, 3D) instead of a slice (two-dimensional, 2D). The volume element (voxel) has equal length in all three axes (x, y and z: isotropic voxel); this is important for reconstruction of images in different planes. To speed up data acquisition (and table movement) it is possible to calculate the attenuation information of one voxel from the detector data of less than one complete rotation (a 180° rotation is enough for a good image).

Anatomy of the Heart by Multislice Computed Tomography.
By Francesco Fulvio Faletra, Natesa G. Pandian and Siew Yen Ho. Published 2008 by Wiley-Blackwell Publishing, ISBN: 978-1-4051-8055-9.

The acquisition time depends on the number of detectors, rotation speed of the tube-detector unit, length of volume examined and speed of table movement.

Post-processing imaging modalities

Axial images
Axial images are the basic generated images used in MSCT. Axial images can be viewed directly for interpretation or used to create multiplanar or 3D images.

Multiplanar reconstruction (MPR)
Multiplanar reconstruction is the process of using data from axial MSCT images to create "non-axial" two-dimensional images. MPR images are generated from a plane of only one voxel in thickness transecting a set of axial images. In principle any plane can be generated from the volume data set but, by convention, the most used planes are the body planes (axial, sagittal and coronal) (see Chapter 2). Cardiac planes (parallel to the long axis of the left ventricle) are useful to evaluate the heart anatomy, and oblique planes (at any angulation) to display individual structures such as mitral leaflets or the aortic root (Fig. 1.2; see also Chapters 2 and 3).

Curved multiplanar reconstruction (cMPR)
This display modality produces a flattened representation of a curved plane. This modality is useful for the visualization of coronary arteries: a cMPR is reconstructed along the curved course of the vessel. All curved structures are represented on a flat plane. Because the plane is defined by the course of the coronary vessel of interest, the anatomical relationships of all other structures around the vessel are distorted (Fig. 1.3).

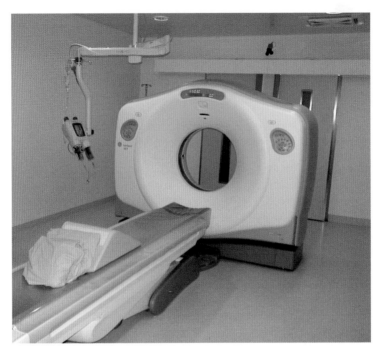

Figure 1.1 A modern multislice computed tomography machine (see text).

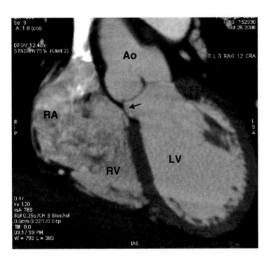

Figure 1.2 Multiplanar reconstruction. An oblique view aims to visualize the membranous septum (arrow). RA = right atrium; RV = right ventricle; Ao = aorta; LV = left ventricle.

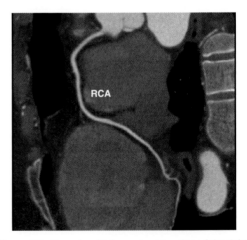

Figure 1.3 Curved multiplanar reconstruction of the right coronary artery (RCA). Although the artery has a tortuous course passing through many planes the algorithm projects the entire course of the vessel in a single plane. Note that the anatomic relationships between chambers are distorted.

Maximum intensity projection (MIP)

With this modality several voxels are stacked one on top of the other, so that slices thicker than one voxel are reconstructed. With MIP, only the voxels with the highest density are visualized. MIP is useful to evaluate small tortuous structures that are hyperdense (i.e., of higher density) compared with their surrounding structures (i.e., contrast-enhanced coronary vessels surrounded by fat). This display modality resembles the images of

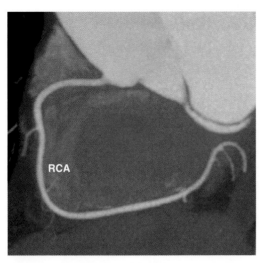

Figure 1.4   The MIP image of the right coronary artery (RCA). This modality is similar to conventional coronary angiography.

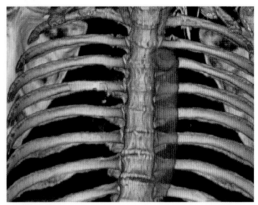

Figure 1.5   The white-yellow color assigned to the ribs makes the image of the chest cage similar to the actual anatomy.

conventional coronary angiography because the result is a projection of the highest attenuation values of the volume (Fig. 1.4).

Volume rendering technique

The 3D volume rendering technique is the computer algorithm used to transform serially acquired axial CT image data into 3D images. Each voxel is classified by calculating the probability that it contains a specific tissue type, with separate classifications for tissues such as bone soft tissue, contrast-enhanced vessels, air, and fat.

By applying color to the histogram tissue classification system, an intuitive perception of depth relationships can be achieved. The application of this "pseudo-color" to tissue classification can be used to enhance discrimination among structures. Although these color schemes (red for soft tissues such as heart and liver, yellow for vessels, white for bones, etc.) do not represent the true optical color of anatomical tissues (the color assignment is arbitrary and tailored for any individual applications), the volume-rendering computer algorithm of the heart displays the heart and great vessels as a nearly perfect copy of the anatomic specimen (Fig. 1.5). One of the strengths of 3D volume rendering is the ability to select a variety of viewing perspectives (Fig. 1.6).

Furthermore, an opacity value can be assigned to each voxel. By increasing or decreasing their opacity values the corresponding voxels become respectively more transparent or more opaque. The opacity setting can be arbitrarily selected according to the requirement of the observer. This display modality is useful for evaluating the coronary tree anatomy and its relationship with encased cavities (Fig. 1.7). Moreover, by making the coronary tree and the myocardium completely transparent and increasing the opacity of the intracavitary contrast, a high-resolution "electronic cast" of the cavities is produced (Fig. 1.8).

Virtual endoscopy

Another modality of imaging called "virtual endoscopy" can be obtained by making the contrast of the cavities transparent and the walls opaque. The viewpoint of the observer is within the cavity and can be moved in any direction. Although the clinical value of this modality in pathological states is not well defined, the comprehensive images are very useful for anatomical purposes (Fig. 1.9).

Endocardial surface modality

In this modality the contrast is made transparent and the endocardial surface of the wall is displayed. Cropping the entire volume data set in any desired planes makes visualization of the endocardial surfaces possible from any perspective (Fig. 1.10).

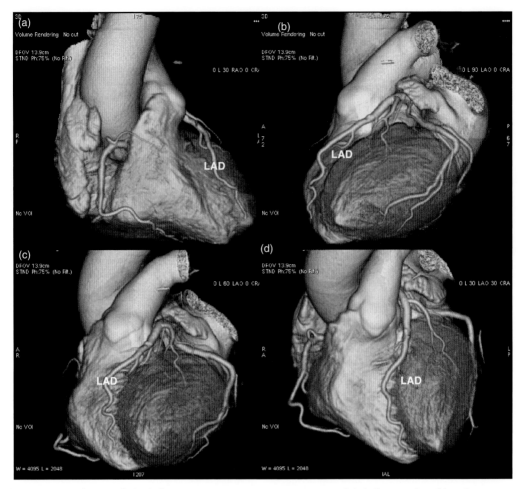

Figure 1.6 3D volume rendering is the most common method of display and assumes external visualization of an object, much like viewing a statue in a museum. 3D display is based on the assumption that light rays reaching our eyes are parallel, similar to seeing objects from a great distance. With this method a countless number of perspectives can be selected (a–d). LAD = left anterior descending coronary artery.

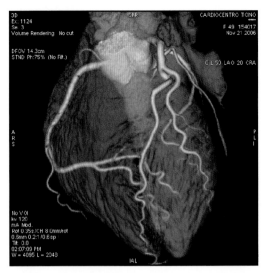

Figure 1.7 By increasing the opacity value of the coronary tree, decreasing the opacity of contrast inside the cavities and making the myocardium completely transparent, clear images of the coronary tree arborization and its relationship with encased cavities can be obtained.

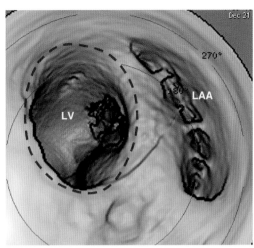

Figure 1.9 Virtual endoscopy. The perspective is inside the left atrium. The mitral valve annulus (red dotted circle), the left ventricle (LV) as well as the left atrial appendage (LAA) can be seen. Rather than light rays being parallel, projected light rays are focused to converge on the viewpoint, simulating natural light convergence on the human retina. The resulting distortion facilitates perception of distance on the basis of object size. Objects near the viewpoint appear large, whereas objects farther away appear small.

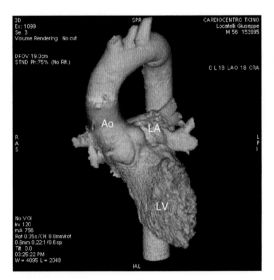

Figure 1.8 "Electronic casts" of the left heart cavities. The relationships between cavities are easily appreciated. LV = left ventricle; LA = left atrium; Ao = aorta.

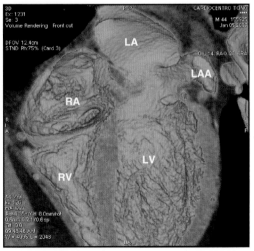

Figure 1.10 3D endocardial surface modality. The posterior endocardial surfaces of right atrium (RA), right ventricle (RV), left atrium (LA) and left ventricle (LV) are displayed viewed from an antero-superior perspective. LAA = left atrial appendage.

Suggested reading

Calhoun PS, Kuszyk BS, Heath DG, Carley JC, Fishman EK. Three-dimensional volume rendering of spiral CT data: theory and method. *RadioGraphics* 1999;19:745–776.

Cody DD. AAPM/RSNA physics tutorial for residents: topics in CT. *RadioGraphics* 2002;22:1255–1268.

Fishman EK, Drebin B, Magid D *et al*. Volumetric rendering techniques: applications for three dimensional imaging of the hip. *Radiology* 1987;163:737–738.

Van Ooijen PM, Ho KY, Dorgelo J, Oudkerk M. Coronary artery imaging with multidetector CT: visualization issues. *RadioGraphics* 2003;23:e16.

CHAPTER 2

Location of the Heart: Body Planes and Axis

Location of the heart

The heart is positioned within the mediastinum with one-third of its mass to the right of the midline, and with its own long axis directed from the right shoulder towards the left hip (Fig. 2.1a–d). It is bordered bilaterally by the lungs, anteriorly by the sternum and inferiorly by the diaphragm. The cardiac apex is located in the left hemithorax (Fig. 2.2a–d).

The right border of the silhouette, more or less vertical, is produced by the right atrium, with the caval veins entering at its top and bottom. The inferior border is made by the right ventricle, extending horizontally along the diaphragm to the cardiac apex, with the left border sloping upwards from the apex and formed by the wall of the left ventricle. At the top of the left border, the left atrial appendage contributes to the silhouette. The pulmonary trunk and aorta emerge from the superior border of the silhouette, with the aorta in a rightward position (Fig. 2.3).

The right heart is located anteriorly and the left heart posteriorly. The right heart structures (right ventricular infundibulum and pulmonary trunk) are therefore anterior relative to the left heart and not located directly to the right (Figs. 2.1a–d and 2.2a–d). The right ventricle is the most anteriorly situated cardiac chamber, lying behind the sternum (Figs. 2.1d and 2.2a). The atrial chambers are

Anatomy of the Heart by Multislice Computed Tomography.
By Francesco Fulvio Faletra, Natesa G. Pandian and
Siew Yen Ho. Published 2008 by Wiley-Blackwell Publishing,
ISBN: 978-1-4051-8055-9.

posterior and to the right of their respective ventricular chambers (Figs. 2.1d and 2.2d).

Furthermore, owing to the curvature of the ventricular septum, the outflow tract of the right ventricle sweeps antero-superiorly relative to that of the left ventricular outflow tract (Fig. 2.4a,b). The aortic root is thus centrally located in the heart. From its rightward position, the ascending aorta curves leftward to continue into the aortic arch, which passes to the left of the trachea and descends posteriorly as the thoracic aorta. The aortic arch is superior to the bifurcation of the pulmonary trunk (Fig. 2.5a,b).

The most anterior part of the left ventricle is the septum, which includes more than 40% of the cardiac mass. The anterior wall (A) of the left ventricle is actually superior, with the lateral wall lying superior and posterior (L), and the posterior wall inferior-posterior (P). Accordingly the "left anterior descending coronary artery" is superior and the "posterior" descending coronary artery is inferior (Fig. 2.6).

Body planes

Multislice computed tomography (MSCT) images are digital, and more than 1000 axis images are generated by the latest MSCT machines. Any slice has three dimensions: the width (x-axis), the height (y-axis) and the thickness (z-axis). Any slice is therefore divided into "voxels" (volume elements). In the modern MSCT the shape of voxels approximates closely to a small cube (isotropic, i.e., the x-, y-, and z-axes are almost equal). The volume data set of any MSCT examination consists of millions of voxels (Fig. 2.7).

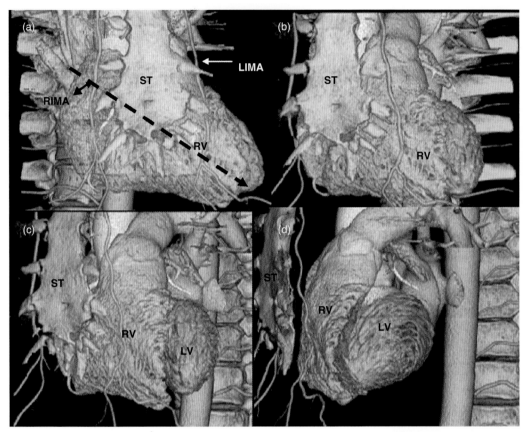

Figure 2.1 (a–d) Electronic cast showing the position of the heart in the thorax. Views from anterior (a) to left lateral (d) perspective. See text and Video clip 1, Position of the heart (Lateral rotation) 👁. RV = right ventricle; LV = left ventricle; ST = sternum; LIMA = left internal mammary artery; RIMA = right internal mammary artery.

In principle, any plane can be generated from this huge volume data set. However, by convention and with the subject standing in an upright position and facing the observer, three orthogonal planes are usually derived: sagittal, coronal and axial. For the body, two of these planes are in the long axis (sagittal and coronal), whereas the axial plane is transverse and in the short axis.

Axial planes

An axial plane divides the body into top and bottom portions (Figs. 2.8 and 2.9). These sections taken "from the head to the feet" usually produce a family of oblique cross-sections of the heart with truncated or expanded views of chambers and walls because of the oblique position of the heart within the thorax. Some of the transverse views appear similar to the echocardiographic short-axis views. Transverse sectioning at the level of the great arteries provides an anatomic display of the pulmonary trunk and its bifurcation into the right and left main pulmonary arteries and an adjacent cross-section of the ascending aorta. Moreover, from this plane the origins of the left and right coronary arteries can be appreciated (Fig. 2.10).

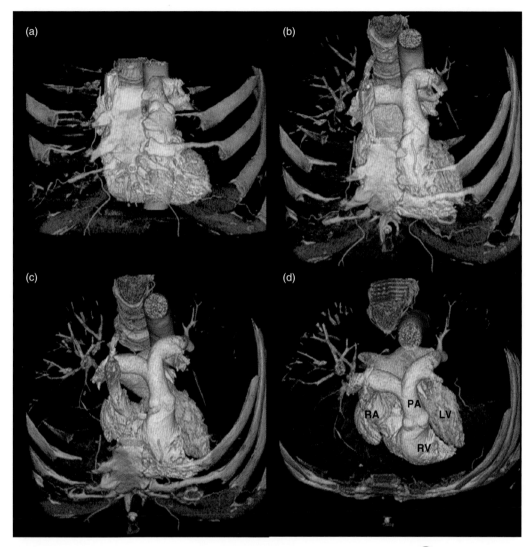

Figure 2.2 Electronic cast (see also Video clip 2, Position of the heart (supero-inferior rotation) 👁). (a–d) Views from anterior (a) to above (d). RV = right ventricle; LV = left ventricle; RA = right atrium; PA = pulmonary artery.

Sagittal planes

The sagittal plane divides the body into right and left sides. Structures lying within different parts of the sagittal plane are then said to be anterior or posterior relative to each other (Figs. 2.11 and 2.12). The slices of the sagittal plane run from right to left or vice versa. This plane is useful for imaging the right ventricle outflow tract and the descending thoracic aorta (Fig. 2.13). Whenever the long axis of the left ventricle is horizontal, for example, in obese patients, the sagittal plane may be useful for imaging short axis views of the left ventricle.

Coronal planes

The coronal plane divides the body into front and back sections. Structures lying within different parts of the sagittal plane are then described as

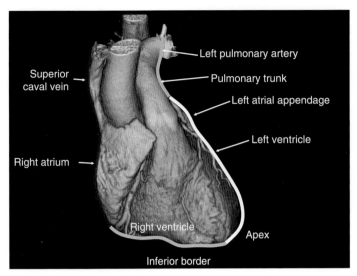

Figure 2.3 3D volume rendering. The cardiac silhouette (see text).

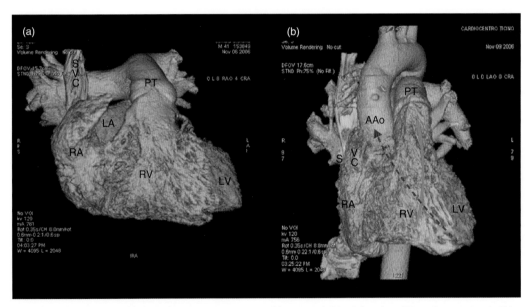

Figure 2.4 Electronic cast. (a) The right structures are anterior relative to the left structures. (b) The outflow tract of the right ventricle sweeps antero-superiorly relative to the left ventricular outflow tract (red and blue arrows). LA = left atrium; PT = pulmonary trunk; RV = right ventricle; LV = left ventricle; AAo = ascending aorta; RA = right atrium; SVC = superior vena cava.

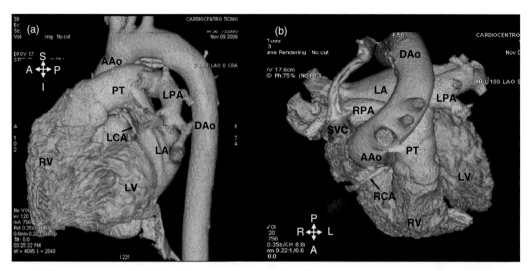

Figure 2.5 (a,b) Electronic cast showing the course of the aorta relative to the pulmonary trunk (see text). Note in this patient the right coronary artery (RCA) origins from the left Valsava sinus. PT = pulmonary trunk; RV = right ventricle; LV = left ventricle; LA = left atrium; AAo = ascending aorta; DAo = descending aorta; RPA = right pulmonary artery; LPA = left pulmonary artery; LCA = left circumflex artery.

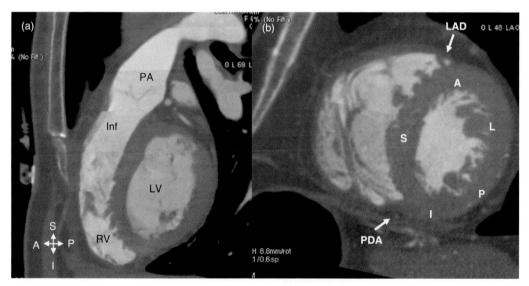

Figure 2.6 Axial (a) and short-axis (b) section showing the right ventricle as anterior and the left ventricle posterior, the anterior wall (A) superior, the lateral wall (L) superior-posterior and the posterior wall (P) inferior-posterior (I). The left anterior descending coronary artery (LAD) is actually superior and the posterior descending coronary artery (PDA) is inferior. RV = right ventricle; LV = left ventricle; PA = pulmonary artery; Inf = infundibulum.

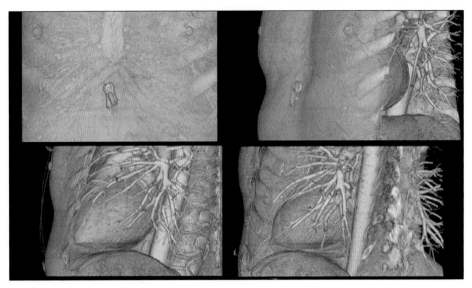

Figure 2.7   3D volume rendering. Volume data set of a patient who underwent CT coronary angiography. This data set comprises millions of voxels (see text and Video clip 3, Thorax).

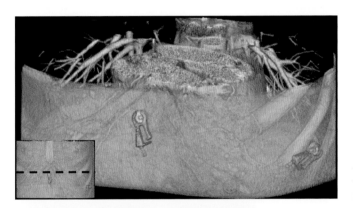

Figure 2.8   3D volume rendering. Axial view. The heart and thorax are cut along the axial plane. The inset shows the plane of the cut.

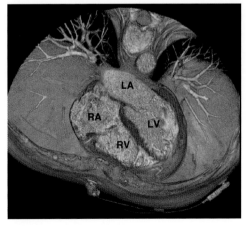

Figure 2.9   3D volume rendering. Axial view; perspective from above. LA = left atrium; LV = left ventricle; RA = right atrium; RV = right ventricle.

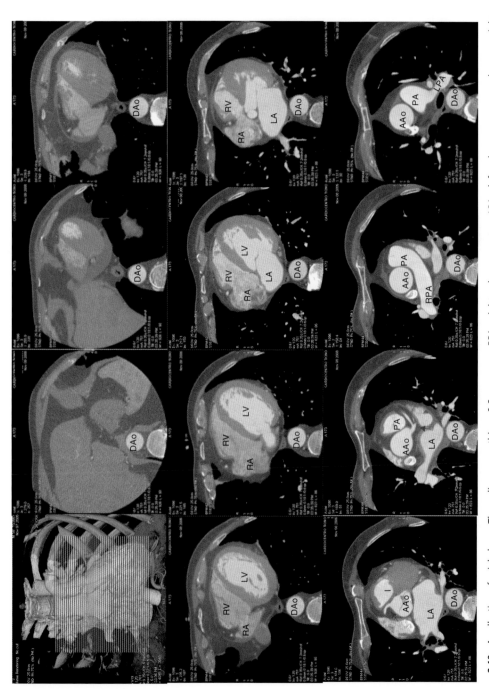

Figure 2.10 A collection of axial planes. These slices are as thin as 0.6 mm. PA = pulmonary artery; RA = right atrium; RV = right ventricle; LV = left ventricle; LA = left atrium; AAo = ascending aorta; DAo = descending aorta; RPA = right pulmonary artery; LPA = left pulmonary artery; red arrow = right and left coronary artery; I = infundibulum.

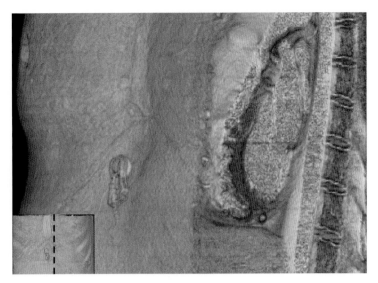

Figure 2.11 3D volume rendering. Axial view. The heart and thorax are cut along the sagittal plane. The inset shows the plane of the cut.

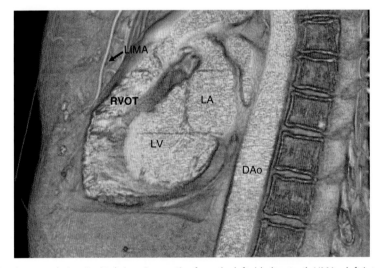

Figure 2.12 3D volume rendering. Sagittal view. Perspective from the left side (see text). LIMA = left internal mammary artery; RVOT = right ventricle outflow tract; LV = left ventricle; LA = left atrium; DAo = descending aorta.

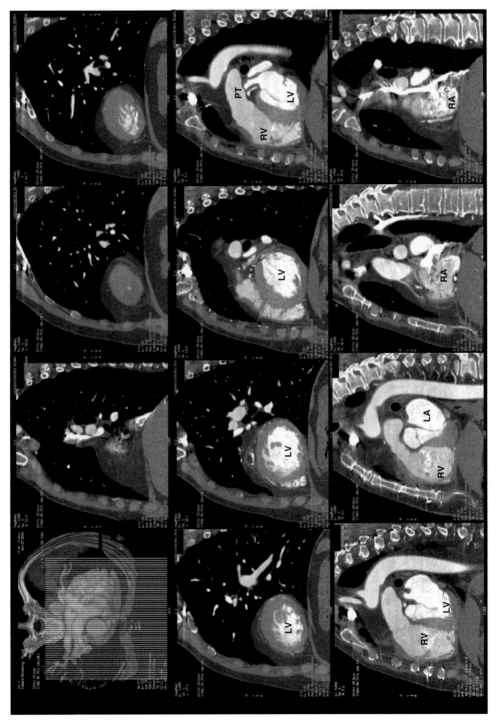

Figure 2.13   A collection of sagittal planes. Abbreviations as in previous figures.

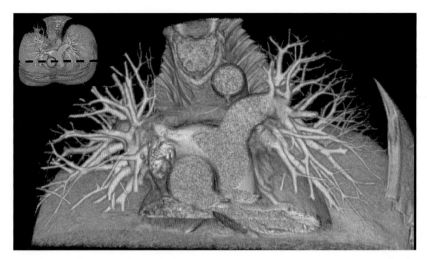

Figure 2.14   3D volume rendering. Axial view. The heart and thorax are cut along the coronal plane. The figure in the upper left corner shows the plane of the cut.

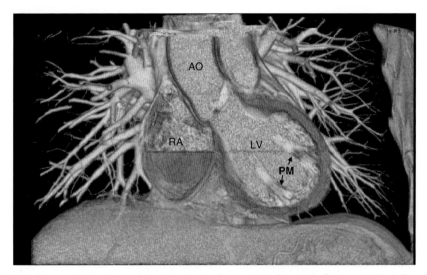

Figure 2.15   3D volume rendering. Coronal view. Perspective from anterior (see text). AO = aorta; LV = left ventricle; RA = right atrium; PM = papillary muscles.

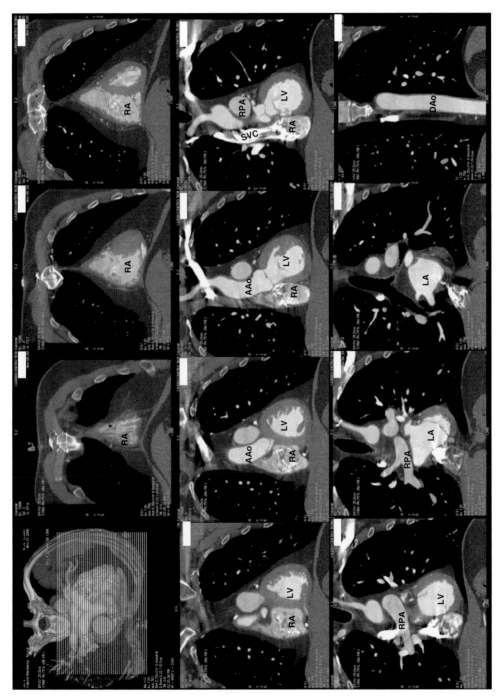

Figure 2.16 A collection of coronal planes. Abbreviations as in previous figures.

being right and left relative to each other (Figs. 2.14 and 2.15). Accordingly, the slices run from anterior to posterior and vice versa. Coronal planes are best for imaging the left ventricular outflow tract, aortic valve and descending thoracic aorta (Fig. 2.16).

Suggested reading

Anderson RH, Becker AE. *Cardiac Anatomy*. Edinburgh: Churchill Livingstone, 1980.

Anderson RH, Ho SY, Brecker SJ. Anatomic basis of cross-sectional echocardiography. *Heart* 2001;85:716–720.

Anderson RH, Razavi R, Taylor AM. Cardiac anatomy revisited. *J Anat* 2004;205:159–177.

Cosio FG, Anderson RH, Kuck KH *et al*. Living anatomy of the atrioventricular junctions. A guide to electrophysiologic mapping. A Consensus Statement from the Cardiac Nomenclature Study Group, Working Group of Arrhythmias, European Society of Cardiology, and the Task Force on Cardiac Nomenclature from NASPE. *Circulation* 1999;100:e31–e37.

McAlpine WA. Heart and Coronary Arteries. Berlin: Springer-Verlag, 1975.

CHAPTER 3

Cardiac Planes

Orthogonal views along the body planes are useful for evaluating the overall morphology of the heart. However, because these planes are not perpendicular to the wall or cavities, cardiac imaging planes are needed. These are the planes through the heart's long and short axes.

Three main long-axis views of the left ventricle oriented parallel to the long axis of the left ventricle are usually used (Figs. 3.1–3.4). These views are the long-axis view and the four- and two-chamber views. The long-axis view cuts through the anterior portion of the septum and the posterior left ventricular wall thus including both the inflow and outflow tracts of the left ventricle (Fig. 3.5a,b). This plane also cuts obliquely through the right ventricular outflow. As in an echocardiographic parasternal or apical long-axis view, the aortic valve with the right and non-coronary sinuses and the mid-portion of anterior (aortic) and posterior (mural) mitral leaflets are displayed. The posterior-medial papillary muscle can be well demonstrated. The upper and lower left pulmonary veins enter the roof of the left atrium (Fig. 3.5a, arrows). Finally, the proximal portion of the right coronary artery in cross-sectional view is also imaged.

The four-chamber plane cuts the heart along both lateral walls from the apex to base so that both ventricles and atria are included in the plane of section (Fig. 3.6a,b). As in echocardiography the

four-chamber view displays the inflow chamber of the left and right ventricles, the mid-posterior septum and the left and right lateral walls. Usually this cut offsets papillary muscles, which are located in different planes. The so-called atrioventricular septum is easily imaged from this view (see Chapter 7 regarding septa). The left and right lower pulmonary veins can be seen (Fig. 3.6a, arrows). The mitral and tricuspid valves are also well demonstrated. The mid-portion of right coronary artery in cross axis view is imaged.

The two-chamber view mirrors the echocardiographic apical and transesophageal two-chamber view (Fig. 3.7a,b). The two-chamber view is obtained by cutting the heart immediately to the left of the ventricular septum from the left ventricular apex through the left mitral orifice and the left atrium (Fig. 3.3). The left anterior descending artery can be displayed in 3D volume rendering along its course in the interventricular sulcus (Fig. 3.7a). This section cuts the anterior and inferior walls. The posterior papillary muscle is usually depicted. The posterior course of the right coronary artery, in patients with right coronary dominance, and the coronary sinus (Fig. 3.7b) are visualized in cross-section. Finally, the section cuts the left atrial appendage.

Figure 3.8 shows the short-axis views of the heart. Short-axis cuts are oriented at 90° relative to the long axis of the left ventricle through the middle of the ventricle. They show the crescentic right ventricle and the circular left ventricle. The aorta and pulmonary trunk as well as left and right atria can be imaged in more cranial cuts (Figs. 3.9 and 3.10).

Anatomy of the Heart by Multislice Computed Tomography. By Francesco Fulvio Faletra, Natesa G. Pandian and Siew Yen Ho. Published 2008 by Wiley-Blackwell Publishing, ISBN: 978-1-4051-8055-9.

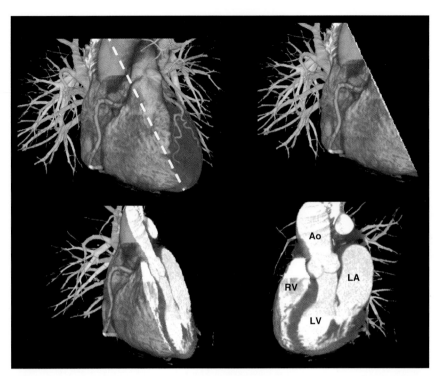

Figure 3.1   3D volume rendering. The heart is cut to show the long-axis view. RV = right ventricle; LA = left atrium; LV = left ventricle; Ao = aorta.

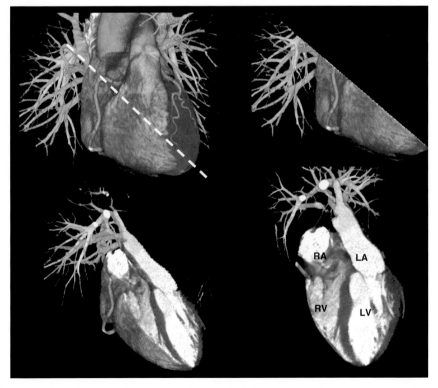

Figure 3.2   3D volume rendering. The heart is cut to show the four-chamber view. RA = right atrium; RV = right ventricle; LA = left atrium; LV = left ventricle.

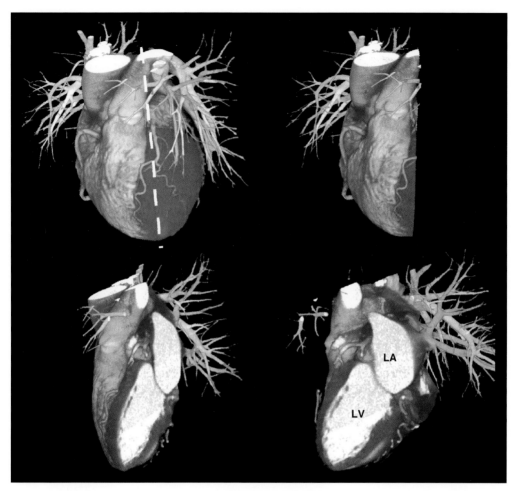

Figure 3.3 3D volume rendering. The heart is cut to show the two-chamber view. LA = left atrium; LV = left ventricle.

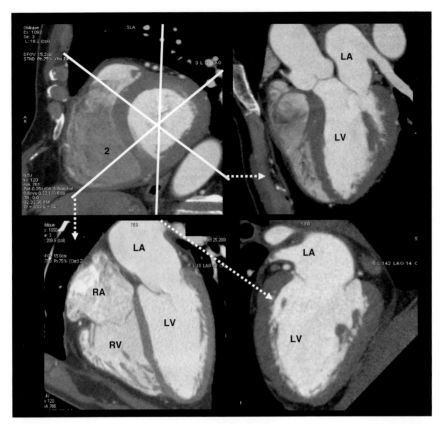

Figure 3.4   The three main long-axis planes. LA = left atrium; LV = left ventricle; RA = right atrium; RV = right ventricle.

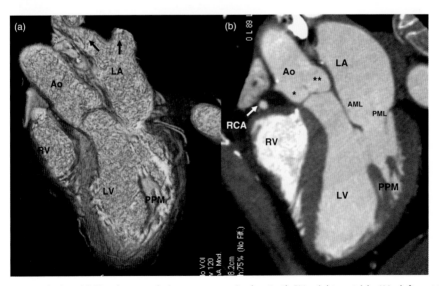

Figure 3.5   Long-axis view. (a) 3D volume rendering reconstruction and (b) the corresponding plane. The single and double asterisks in panel b mark the right and the non-coronary cusps. The arrows in panel a mark the upper and the lower left pulmonary veins (see text). RV = right ventricle; LV = left ventricle; LA = left atrium; Ao = aorta; PPM = posterior papillary muscle; RCA = right coronary artery; AML = anterior mitral leaflet; PML = posterior mitral leaflet.

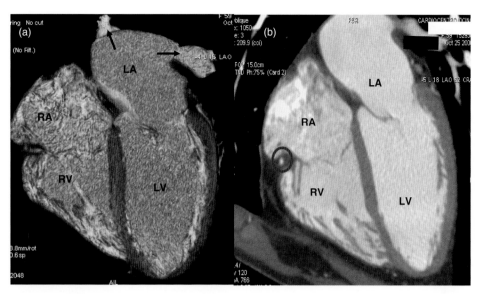

Figure 3.6 Four-chamber view. (a) 3D volume rendering reconstruction and (b) the corresponding plane. Arrows in panel a mark the left and right lower pulmonary veins. The right coronary artery is seen in cross section (red circle in panel b) (see text). RA = right atrium; RV = right ventricle; LA = left atrium; LV = left ventricle.

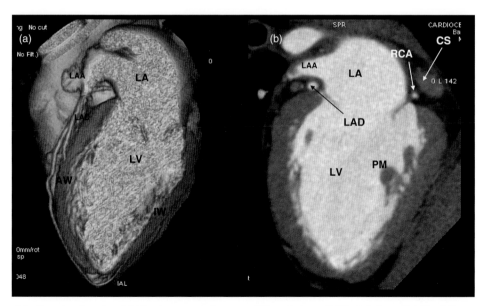

Figure 3.7 Two-chamber view. (a) 3D volume rendering reconstruction and (b) the corresponding plane (see text). LAA = left atrial appendage; LV = left ventricle; AW = anterior wall; IW = inferior wall; LAD = left anterior descending artery; RCA = right coronary artery; CS = coronary sinus; PM = papillary muscle.

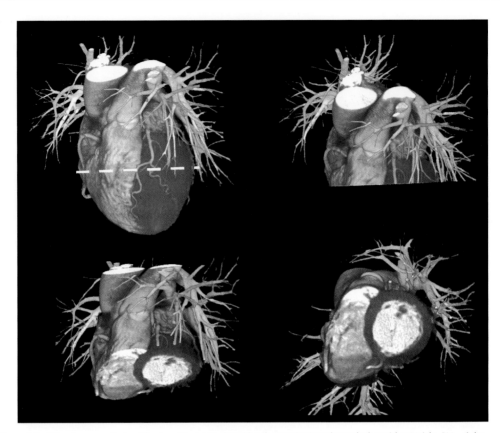

Figure 3.8   3D volume rendering. The heart is cut to show the short-axis view through the mid-ventricle. RV = right ventricle; LV = left ventricle.

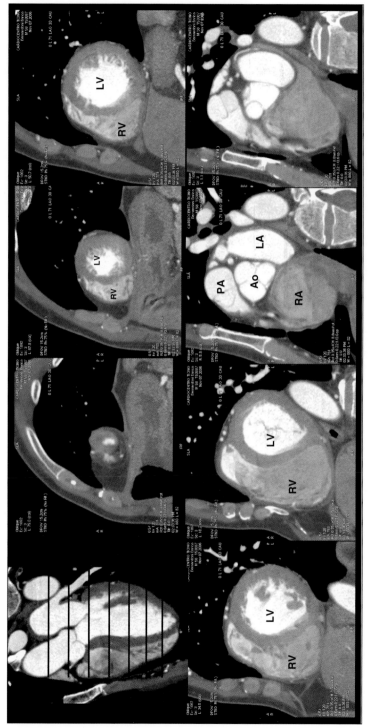

Figure 3.9 A collection of short-axis views from the apex to the base. RV = right ventricle; LV = left ventricle; RA = right atrium; LA = left atrium; Ao = aorta; PA = pulmonary artery.

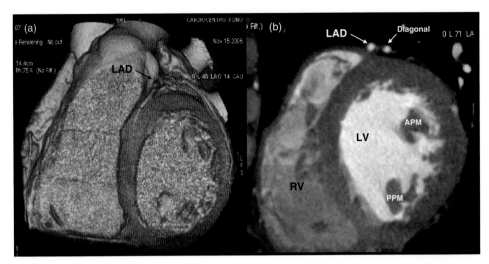

Figure 3.10   Short-axis view at the level of papillary muscles. 3D volume rendering reconstruction (a) and the corresponding oblique plane (b). Antero-lateral (APM) and postero-medial (PPM) papillary muscles can be imaged. Moreover, the left anterior descending coronary artery (LAD) and a diagonal branch are visualized in cross-section (arrows). RV = right ventricle; LV = left ventricle.

Suggested reading

American Heart Association, American College of Cardiology, and Society of Nuclear Medicine. Standardization of cardiac tomographic imaging. *Circulation* 1992;86:338–339.

Edwards WD, Tajik AJ, Seward JB. Standardized nomenclature and anatomic basis for regional tomographic analysis of the heart. *Mayo Clin Proc* 1981;56:479–497.

Waller BF, Taliercio CP, Slack JD *et al.* Tomographic views of normal and abnormal hearts: the anatomic basis for various cardiac imaging techniques, Part I. *Clin Cardiol* 1990;13:804–812.

Waller BF, Taliercio CP, Slack JD *et al.* Tomographic views of normal and abnormal hearts: the anatomic basis for various cardiac imaging techniques, Part II. *Clin Cardiol* 1990;13:877–884.

CHAPTER 4

The Right Heart

Although termed "right heart," this half of the heart is not located entirely in the right chest nor is it strictly to the right of the "left heart" (see Chapter 2). The "electronic" cast of the right heart, viewed from an anterior perspective, is displayed in Fig. 4.1. It shows the characteristic normal U-shape arrangement with the superior caval vein (superior vena cava) and right atrium forming one limb, the right ventricle forming the bend with its outflow tract (the infundibulum) and the pulmonary trunk forming the other limb. With this arrangement, the two valves in the right heart do not abut each other. Instead, a fold of muscle, the ventriculo-infundibular fold, interposes between the tricuspid and pulmonary valves (Figs. 4.1 and 4.2).

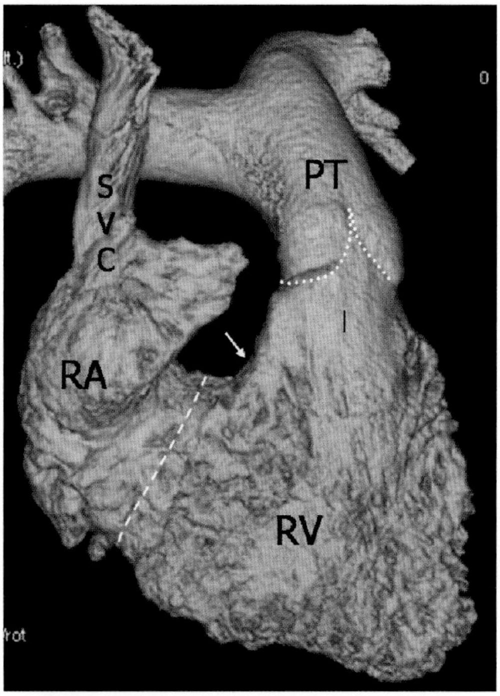

Right atrium

The right atrium comprises a venous component, an appendage, and a vestibular portion that leads to the orifice of the tricuspid valve. The venous component receives the superior (SVC) and inferior caval veins. It forms the posterior wall of the right atrium (Fig. 4.3). The junction between the appendage and the venous component is marked on the epicardial aspect by the sulcus terminalis (terminal groove) (Fig. 4.4), which is usually filled with fatty tissue. The sulcus corresponds to a muscular crest named the crista terminalis (terminal crest) on the endocardial surface. This is a prominent

Figure 4.1 The "electronic" cast of the right heart. Anterior perspective. Superior vena cava (SVC), right atrium (RA), right ventricle (RV), infundibulum (I) and pulmonary trunk (PT) form a U-shaped structure. The ventriculo-infundibular fold (arrow) separates the right heart valves (broken lines).

muscular band that separates the smooth wall of the venous component from the rough wall of the atrial appendage (Fig. 4.5). The crista terminalis is a roughly C-shaped band that originates from the antero-medial wall of the right atrium, passes along the anterior border of the superior cavo-atrial junction, sweeps laterally and descends toward the entrance of the inferior caval vein

Anatomy of the Heart by Multislice Computed Tomography.
By Francesco Fulvio Faletra, Natesa G. Pandian and Siew Yen Ho. Published 2008 by Wiley-Blackwell Publishing, ISBN: 978-1-4051-8055-9.

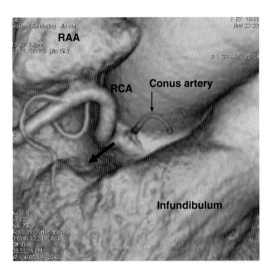

Figure 4.2 3D volume rendering showing the ventriculo-infundibular fold (arrow). View from above and right. Note the conus artery originating independently from the aorta. RAA = right atrial appendage; RCA = right coronary artery.

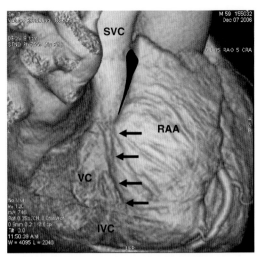

Figure 4.4 3D volume rendering. Postero-lateral view of the right atrium showing the superior (SVC) and inferior (IVC) venae cavae, the venous component (VC) and the right atrial appendage (RAA). Arrows point to the sulcus terminalis. The black-filled shape represents the location of the sinus node.

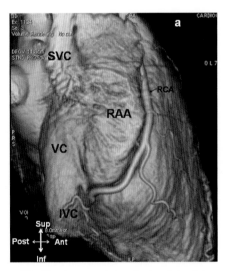

Figure 4.3 3D volume rendering. Postero-lateral view of the right atrium showing the superior (SVC) and inferior (IVC) venae cavae, the venous component (VC) and the right atrial appendage (RAA). RCA = right coronary artery.

(Fig. 4.6). It is of variable thickness and breadth. When cut in cross-section, the muscular band appears like a bump protruding into the atrial cavity (Fig. 4.5c,d). The cephalad portion of the sinus node, the cardiac pacemaker, is located in the antero-superior part of the crista terminalis whereas its tail portion descends within the musculature of the band (Fig. 4.4). In the right anterior oblique view (RAO), the crista terminalis marks the right atrial border (Fig. 4.7). The appendage of the right atrium is triangular and has a broad junction with the atrial chamber. Antero-medially, the appendage protrudes from the right atrium and overlaps the aortic root (Fig. 4.8). On the endocardial aspect, the wall of the appendage is lined with pectinate muscles. These bundles emerge in branching fashion from the crista terminalis, terminating at the vestibule. Because the right atrial appendage is a large part of the atrium, the pectinate muscles are distributed extensively (Figs. 4.9 and 4.10).

The vestibule is the portion of the atrium lying immediately proximal to the orifice of the tricuspid valve. Characteristically it is smooth walled. Its distal margin is marked circumferentially by the hingeline (annulus) of the valvar leaflets (Fig. 4.11).

The segment of the vestibule that is located inferiorly on RAO view (see Fig. 4.7) is part of the cavotricuspid isthmus (Fig. 4.12). The inferior isthmus is recognized by electrophysiologists as the region

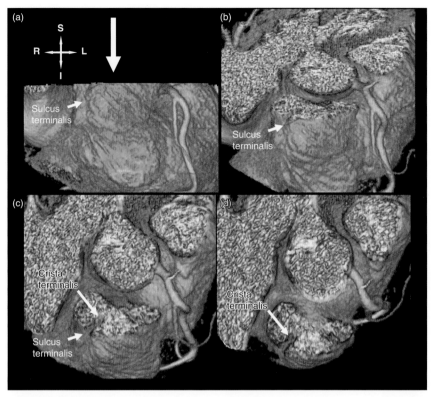

Figure 4.5 (a–d) 3D volume rendering. The data set has been properly cropped and rotated to show the sulcus and the crista terminalis (arrows; see Video clip 4, Right atrium 👁).

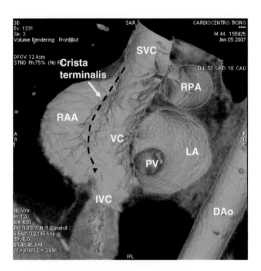

Figure 4.6 3D endocardial perspective showing the C-shaped crista terminalis (dotted line). SVC = superior vena cava; IVC = inferior vena cava; RAA = right atrial appendage; LA = left atrium; PV = pulmonary vein; RPA = right pulmonary artery; DAo = descending aorta; VC = venous component.

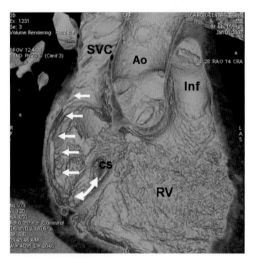

Figure 4.7 3D endocardial surface modality. Right anterior oblique view. The crista terminalis marks the right border of the atrium. The double white arrow marks the region of the inferior isthmus. SVC = superior vena cava; Ao = aorta; RV = right ventricle; Inf = infundibulum; CS = coronary sinus.

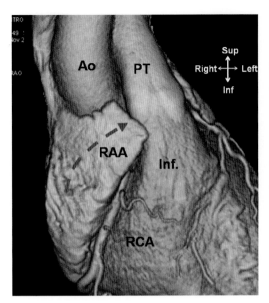

Figure 4.8 The right atrial appendage (RAA) overlaps (red dotted line) the aortic root (Ao) when the heart is viewed from the front. RCA = right coronary artery; Inf = infundibulum; PT = pulmonary trunk.

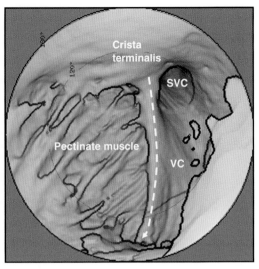

Figure 4.10 Virtual endoscopy. The crista terminalis (dotted line) and the pectinate muscles are clearly visible. SVC = superior vena cava; VC = venous component.

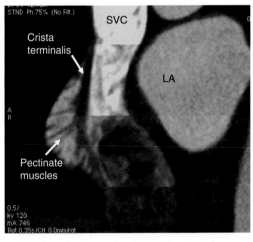

Figure 4.9 A slice image showing pectinate muscles. These muscles originate as branching fibers that emerge at right angles from the terminal crest. SVC = superior vena cava; LA = left atrium.

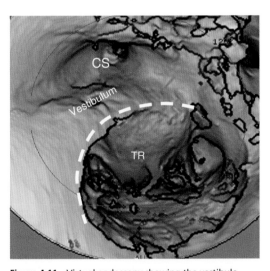

Figure 4.11 Virtual endoscopy showing the vestibule between the ostium of coronary sinus (CS) and the tricuspid annulus (dotted line).

that is ablated to interrupt the circuit of common atrial flutter.

Superiorly, on the septal aspect lies the triangle of Koch with the atrioventricular node toward its apex (Fig. 4.13a,b). A thin fibrous cord known as the tendon of Todaro runs within the musculature of the sinus septum, from the insertion of the eustachian valve, to reach the central fibrous body. The course of the tendon marks the posterior border of the nodal triangle, which is the anatomic landmark for the location of the atrioventricular node of the cardiac conduction system. The anterior border is marked by the hingeline of the septal leaflet whereas the inferior border is the orifice of the coronary sinus together with the vestibule (Fig. 4.13b).

Right ventricle

The right ventricle is the most anteriorly situated cardiac chamber, lying directly behind the sternum.

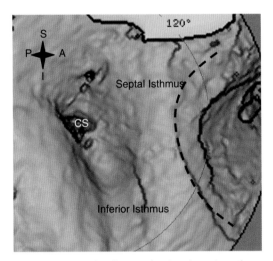

Figure 4.12 Virtual endoscopy showing the ostium of coronary sinus (CS), the annulus of the tricuspid valve (dotted line) and the septal isthmus and inferior isthmus.

The right ventricle's cavity is therefore anterior, overlapping much of the left ventricle (Fig. 4.14). Most of the inferior border of the frontal roentgenogram view of the heart consists of the right ventricle. The right ventricle can be identified externally by its pyramidal shape (Fig. 4.15). When seen from the cardiac apex, the right edge of the right ventricle is a sharp angle, forming the acute margin of the heart (Fig. 4.16). The right ventricle sweeps antero-cephalad to "wrap around" the left ventricle (Fig. 4.17). Viewed from the diaphragmatic aspect of the heart, the right and left ventricles can be seen to lie side by side. The term "crux" of the heart (crux cordis) refers to the intersection between the planes of the atrial and ventricular septa upon the inferior atrioventricular junction. Because the left atrioventricular junction is at not at the same level as the right atrioventricular junction, the crux is not a perfect cross (Fig. 4.18). In the normal heart the wall of the right ventricle is considerably thinner than that of the left ventricle. It ranges in thickness from 3 to 7 mm. At the tip of the apex, however, the wall is particularly thin (Fig. 4.19). The internal appearance of the right ventricle is typical. The shape of the cavity can be imaged as an open "V" with a wide muscular separation between tricuspid and pulmonary valves.

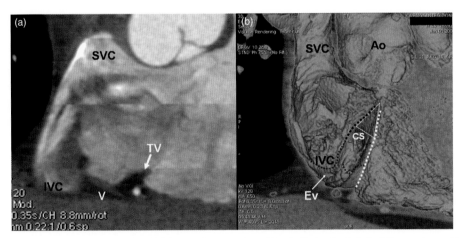

Figure 4.13 (a) Slice image in a simulated right anterior oblique view through the cavo-tricuspid isthmus. Its anterior portion is the smooth vestibular wall (v). (b) The 3D endocardial surface modality shows the eustachian valve (Ev) and coronary sinus (CS). The red triangle marks the location of Koch's triangle. The long red dotted line indicates the inferior isthmus whereas the short red line marks the "septal" isthmus. The white dotted line represents the hingeline of the septal leaflet of the tricuspid valve, and the black dotted line represents the tendon of Todaro, which adjoins the free margin of the eustachian valve (blue dotted line).

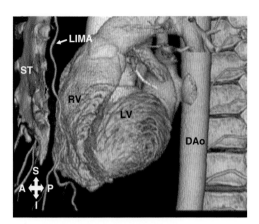

Figure 4.14   Electronic cast. The right ventricle overlaps most of the left ventricle. ST = sternum; RV = right ventricle; LV = left ventricle; LIMA = left internal mammary artery; DAo = descending aorta.

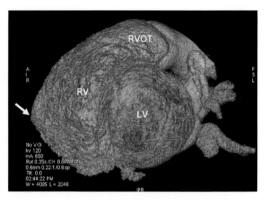

Figure 4.16   Electronic cast viewed from the apex. The arrow marks the acute margin. RV = right ventricle; LV = left ventricle; RVOT = right ventricle outflow tract.

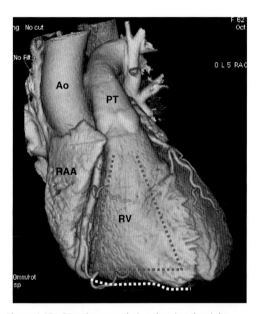

Figure 4.15   3D volume rendering showing the right ventricle. Almost all the inferior border of the frontal view of the heart consists of the right ventricle (dotted white line). The red triangle (dotted red line) illustrates the shape of the right ventricle when viewed from the front. Ao = aorta; PT = pulmonary trunk; RAA = right atrial appendage; RV = right ventricle.

The right ventricle can be divided into three components: the inlet, apical and outlet components (Fig. 4.20).

The most constant characteristic feature of the right ventricle is the presence of coarse apical trabeculations, in contrast to the fine trabeculations found in the left ventricle. In addition, the right ventricle is characterized by the presence of other structures such as (a) the crista supraventricularis (or supraventricular crest), (b) the moderator band and (c) the trabecula septomarginalis (or septomarginal trabeculation) (Fig. 4.21). The crista supraventricularis is the prominent muscular structure that separates tricuspid from pulmonary valves. It comprises the ventriculo-infundibular fold (Fig. 4.21) and its septal insertion into the trabecula septomarginalis. The trabecula septomarginalis is a Y-shaped muscle band that appears like a column supporting the ventriculo-infundibular fold in between its arms (Fig. 4.22). The posterior arm points toward the tricuspid valve and the membranous septum. Deeper cuts into the crista supraventricularis reveal the aortic root and a thin part of the ventricular septum, the membranous septum (Fig. 4.23a,b). Usually, but not always, the body of the Y is adherent to the septum, and in sectional imaging it can appear as a bump on the septum (Fig. 4.24). When abnormally formed or hypertrophied, it can divide the ventricular cavity into two chambers.

The body of the "septomarginal trabeculation" ends near the apex, splitting into several smaller muscle bundles. One of these usually takes a characteristic course crossing the right ventricular cavity. This branch has been named the moderator band because it was thought, wrongly, to limit the diastolic expansion of the chamber (Figs. 4.25 and

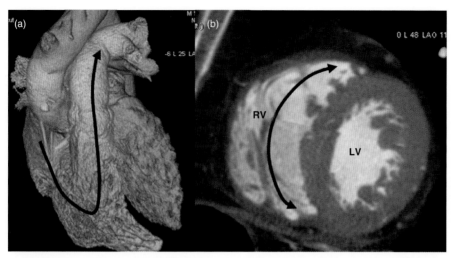

Figure 4.17 (a) The black line in the electronic cast traces the inflow and outflow tracts through the right ventricle. (b) In short-axis view the right ventricle is crescent shaped, curving around the left ventricle. RV = right ventricle; LV = left ventricle.

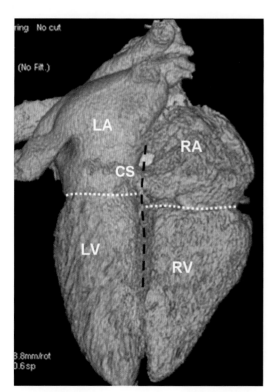

Figure 4.18 Electronic cast of both ventricles. This view from the diaphragmatic aspect shows the course of the coronary sinus (CS) and the cardiac crux, which is the intersection between the plane of the cardiac septa (black broken line) and the inferior atrioventricular junction (white broken lines). RV = right ventricle; LV = left ventricle; RA = right atrium; LA = left atrium.

4.26). The moderator band runs toward the anterior wall, and joins the base of anterior papillary muscle (Fig. 4.27a,b).

The outlet portion of the right ventricle consists of the infundibulum, a circumferential muscular structure that supports the leaflets of the pulmonary valve. Because of the semilunar shape of the pulmonary leaflets, this valve does not have an annulus in the traditional sense of a ring-like attachment. The leaflets have semilunar attachments that cross the musculoarterial junction in a corresponding semilunar fashion (Fig. 4.28a). The outlet component, or infundibulum, is a free-standing and completely muscular structure. The pulmonary valve leaflets are supported entirely by this free-standing musculature. There is an extensive external tissue plane between the walls of the aorta and the pulmonary infundibulum. The leaflets of the pulmonary and aortic valves have markedly different levels of attachments within their respective ventricles. These features allow the pulmonary valve, including its basal attachments within the infundibulum, to be harvested during the Ross procedure without creating a ventricular septal defect (Fig. 4.28b). Another important spatial relationship to note is that the posterior (paraseptal) wall of the infundibulum is in close proximity to the main branches of the coronary arteries (Fig. 4.28).

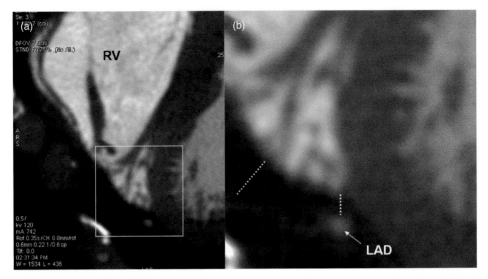

Figure 4.19   The remarkably thin wall of the right ventricle (RV) at its apex (dotted lines) in comparison with the wall nearby. Note the course of the left descending coronary artery (LAD) in cross-section. Figure (b) is the magnified image of figure (a) which is shown as an inset.

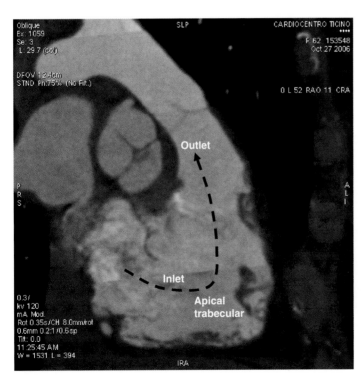

Figure 4.20   A slice image showing the three components of the right ventricle: the inlet, the apical trabecular and the outlet. The dotted line marks the V-shaped cavity. Note the aortic valve imaged in cross-section in the middle.

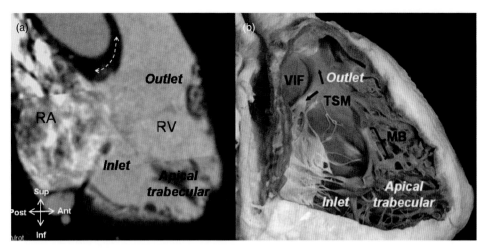

Figure 4.21 (a) A slice image and (b) a specimen showing the inlet, apical trabecular and outlet components of the right ventricle. The ventriculo-infundibular fold (white double-headed arrow; VIF) separates the tricuspid valve from the pulmonary valve. It inserts between the arms (black arrows) of the trabecula septomarginalis (TSM). The moderator band (MB) arises from the TSM and crosses the ventricular chamber as a well-defined muscular bundle to insert into the antero-lateral ventricular wall. The anterior papillary muscle of the tricuspid valve is usually attached to it.

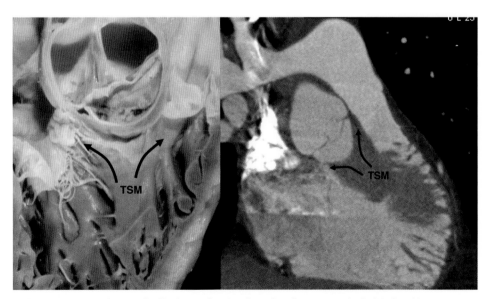

Figure 4.22 Anatomic specimen and a slice image showing the trabecula septomarginalis (TSM) and its arms (arrows).

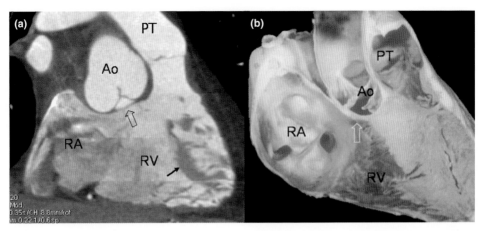

Figure 4.23   (a) This slice cuts into the body of the trabecula septomarginalis (black arrow), the aortic root and the region of thin ventricular septum (open arrow). (b) The heart specimen is displayed in similar orientation but the cut is deeper into the muscular septum and through the thin part of the septum adjacent to the membranous septum (open arrow). Ao = aorta; PT = pulmonary trunk; RA = right atrium; RV = right ventricle.

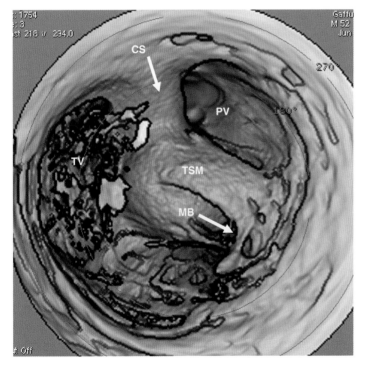

Figure 4.24   3D virtual endoscopy. View from the apex. The crista supraventricularis (CS), the trabecula septomarginalis (TSM) and the moderator band (MB) can be recognized. TV = tricuspid valve; PV = pulmonary valve.

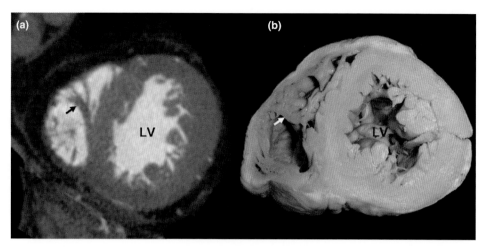

Figure 4.25 Short-axis view (a) and anatomic specimen (b) showing the moderator band (arrow) spanning the septum and the antero-lateral wall of the right ventricle. LV = left ventricle.

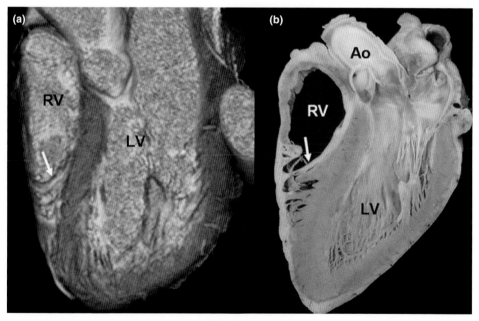

Figure 4.26 (a,b) 3D volume rendering long-axis view and comparable cut of specimen showing the moderator band (arrow). Ao = aorta; LV = left ventricle; RV = right ventricle.

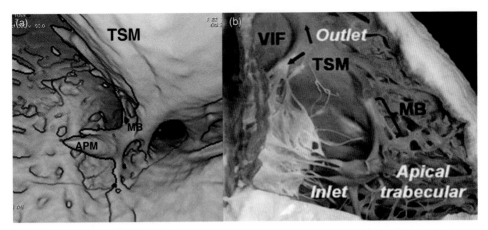

Figure 4.27   (a,b) 3D Virtual endoscopy and anatomic specimen showing the anatomic continuity between the trabecula septomarginalis (TSM), the moderator band (MB) and the anterior papillary muscle (APM). VIF = ventriculo-infundibular fold.

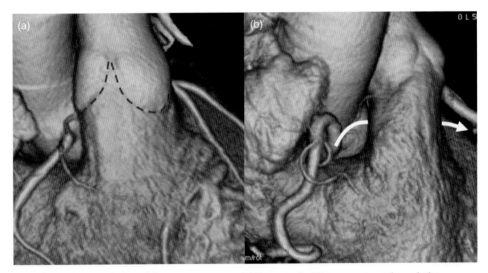

Figure 4.28   (a) 3D volume rendering of the subpulmonary infundibulum and the pulmonary root. The infundibulum elevates the pulmonary valve above the ventricular mass. The crown-shaped hingelines of pulmonary leaflets are indicated by the dotted red lines. (b) The curved white arrow passes through the extracardiac tissue plane between the infundibulum and the aorta. This feature makes it possible to detach the pulmonary valve for use in the surgical Ross procedure without creating a ventricular septal defect.

Suggested reading

Cabrera JA, Sanchez-Quintana D, Farre J, Rubio JA, Ho SY. The inferior right atrial isthmus: further architectural insights for current and coming ablation technologies. *J Cardiovasc Electrophysiol* 2005;16:402–408.

Foale R, Nihoyannopoulos P, McKenna W *et al.* Echocardiographic measurement of the normal adult right ventricle. *Br Heart J* 1986;56:33–44.

Ho SY, Anderson RH, Sanchez-Quintana D. Atrial structure and fibres: morphological basis of atrial conduction. *Cardiovasc Res* 2002;54:325–336.

Ho SY, Nihoyannopoulos P. Anatomy, echocardiography, and normal right ventricular dimensions. *Heart* 2006; 92:2–13.

CHAPTER 5

The Left Heart

Pulmonary veins

Anatomic details of the pulmonary veins, especially at the venous insertions into the left atrium,
have become clinically important owing to the use
of catheter ablation in treating patients with atrial
fibrillation. The pulmonary veins are considered
to have an important role in initiating and main-
taining atrial fibrillation. Current commonly used
ablation strategies aim to isolate the veins from the
left atrium.

The pulmonary veins originate from a capillary
network on the walls of the air sacs, where they
are continuous with the capillary ramifications of
the pulmonary artery. Joining together, they form
one vessel for each lung lobule. These vessels merge
together into a single vein for each lobe – three for
the right lung and two for the left lung. The vein
from the middle lobe of the right lung usually unites
with that from the upper lobe. The most common
pattern is to have two veins from the hilum of each
lung. They open separately into the posterior part
of the left atrium (Fig. 5.1).

The pulmonary vein ostia are the atriopulmonary venous junctions. However, it is often not
possible to identify the precise location of the junctions especially when the veins are funnel-shaped
and have a gradual "entrance" to the atrium. Multislice computed tomography can provide clearer
anatomic delineation thereby reducing the risk of
ablating within the vein and causing venous stenosis. Ablating within the right superior pulmonary
vein also increases the risk of injuring the right

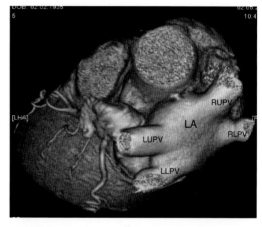

Figure 5.1 3D volume rendering. External view of the
four pulmonary veins and their atriopulmonary junctions.
LUPV = left upper pulmonary vein; LLPV = left lower
pulmonary vein; RUPV = right upper pulmonary vein;
RLPV = right lower pulmonary vein.

phrenic nerve. There are many variants from the
usual pattern of four pulmonary veins. For example, the right hilum may have three veins when the
upper and middle lobes drain independently. Not
infrequently, the veins on the left or the right, or
both sides, join together into a common vein (or
veins) before entering the left atrium. The common segment is often very short and described
as the antrum. On gross examination, it is not
clear where the atriopulmonary venous junction
lies precisely in these hearts. The venous ostia
are ellipsoidal rather than round, with greater
superior–inferior dimensions than antero-posterior
dimensions (Fig. 5.2).

The distal or central pulmonary veins are the
portions of the pulmonary veins in proximity to the left atrium. Electrophysiologists name
the pulmonary vein segments between branch

Anatomy of the Heart by Multislice Computed Tomography.
By Francesco Fulvio Faletra, Natesa G. Pandian and
Siew Yen Ho. Published 2008 by Wiley-Blackwell Publishing,
ISBN: 978-1-4051-8055-9.

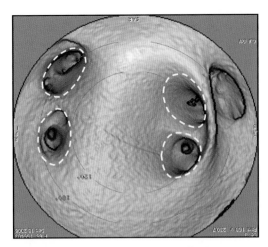

Figure 5.2 Virtual endoscopy. The ostia of pulmonary veins are ellipsoidal with longer superior–inferior dimensions than antero-posterior dimensions.

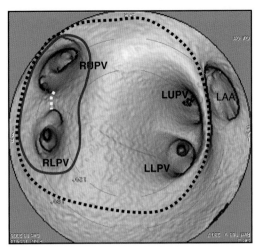

Figure 5.4 Virtual endoscopy. A view from inside looking at the roof of the left atrium. The right intervenous saddle is marked by a white dotted line. The right pulmonary vein inflow vestibule is circled by the solid red line. The black dotted line encircles the whole posterior left atrium. RUPV = right upper pulmonary vein; RLPV = right lower pulmonary vein; LUPV = left upper pulmonary vein; LLPV = left lower pulmonary vein; LAA = left atrial appendage.

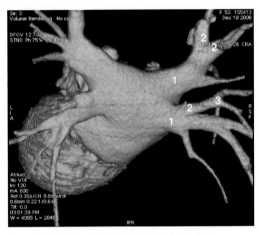

Figure 5.3 Electronic cast. Segments of the distal pulmonary veins from V1 through V3. The V1 segment is the most important segment to include on epicardial views.

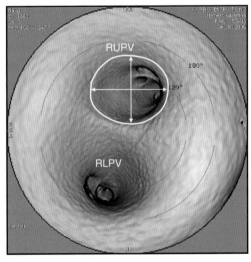

Figure 5.5 Navigator modality. Normal lower and upper veins with the ostial diameters and circumferences measured.

points retrogradely from the atriopulmonary venous junctions. For example, the V1 segment extends retrograde from the ostium to the "first" branch point, which anatomically is the last junction or confluence of branches (Fig. 5.3).

The intervenous "saddle" is the region of atrial wall lying between separate ipsilateral pulmonary veins. The pulmonary vein inflow vestibule includes the ipsilateral pulmonary vein ostia and the intervenous saddle atrial wall. The posterior left atrium includes the bilateral pulmonary vein inflow vestibules and the interposed posterior atrial wall (Figs. 5.4 and 5.5).

On the endocardial aspect, the left atrial wall has a smooth ridge between the entrance of the left

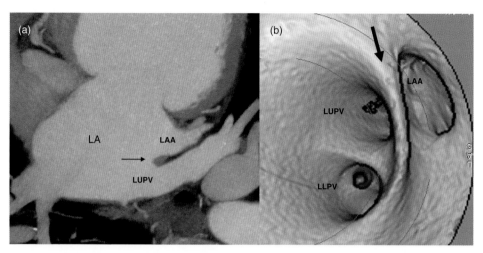

Figure 5.6 (a) Maximum intensity projection (MIP) oblique projection and navigator modality showing a ridge (arrow) projecting into the left atrium (LA). This ridge is caused by an infolding of the wall of the left atrium between the left atrial appendage (LAA) anteriorly and the left upper pulmonary vein (LUPV) posteriorly. (b) A bulbous tip (pointed by arrow) may be misdiagnosed as a mass. LLPV = left lower pulmonary vein.

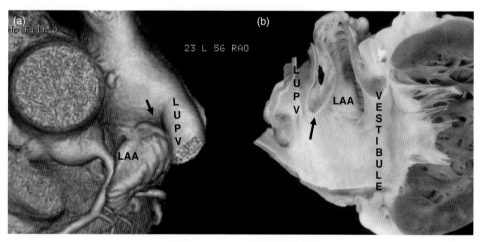

Figure 5.7 (a) 3D volume rendering showing the infolding of the wall of the left atrium (arrow) between the left atrial appendage (LAA) anteriorly and the left upper pulmonary vein (LUPV) posteriorly. (b) The left side of the heart cut longitudinally to show the infolding (arrow) that appears like a ridge on the endocardial surface. The LAA is trabeculated on the endocardial surface whereas the rest of the atrial wall is smooth.

atrial appendage and the ostium of the left superior pulmonary vein. This ridge may have a bulbous tip and can be mistaken for a pedunculated mass or thrombus arising from the lateral wall of the left atrium (Fig. 5.6).

Anatomically, this ridge is an infolding of the wall of the left atrium. Its prominence and width vary considerably (Fig. 5.7) with implications for isolating the atriopulmonary venous junction.

Left atrium

The left atrium is located superiorly and in the midline. It is the most posteriorly situated cardiac

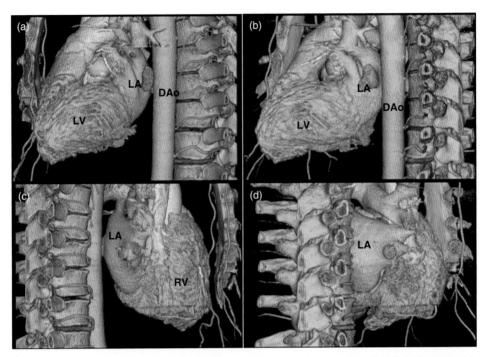

Figure 5.8 3D electronic cast showing the superior–posterior position of left atrium from the left (a,b) and the right and right-posterior (c,d) perspectives. LA = left atrium; LV = left ventricle; DAo = descending aorta; RV = right ventricle.

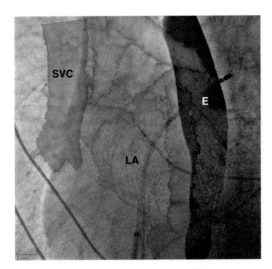

Figure 5.9 "Fusion imaging" between MSCT of the left atrium (LA) and barium swallow of the esophagus (E). SVC = superior vena cava.

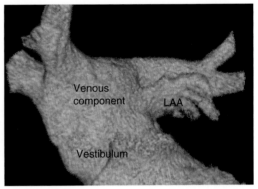

Figure 5.10 Electronic cast of the left atrium. The left atrium, similarly to the right atrium, consists of a smooth-walled venous component that receives the four pulmonary veins, the vestibule and the left atrial appendage (LAA).

chamber. Consequently, its posterior wall is adjacent to the course of the esophagus, separated only by the pericardium (Fig. 5.8).

The descent of the esophagus has a variable relationship with the atrial wall and with the atriopulmonary venous junctions, in the middle, or more to the right or the left. Delineation of the location of the esophagus can help reduce the risk of causing atrioesophageal fistulas when carrying out ablations for atrial fibrillation (Fig. 5.9).

Like the right atrium, the left atrium consists of three components: the appendage, vestibule,

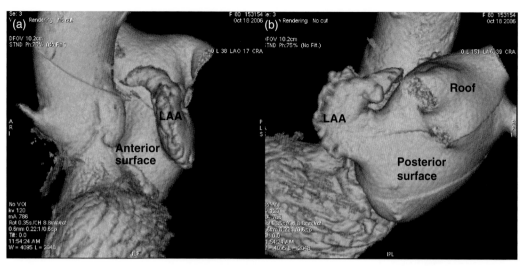

Figure 5.11   Electronic cast showing the anterior (a), the posterior surfaces and the roof (b) of the left atrium. LAA = left atrial appendage.

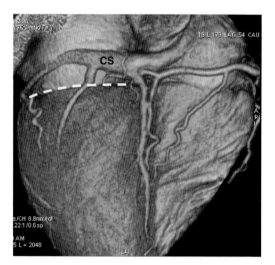

Figure 5.12   3D volume rendering of the posterior aspect of the heart. The coronary sinus (CS) runs superiorly from the level of the mitral valve hingeline.

and venous component. It is mainly smooth walled because its venous component is considerably larger than the appendage. The smooth wall continues into the vestibule that surrounds the atrial outlet, leading to the mitral valve (Figs. 5.10 and 5.11).

Related to the epicardial aspect of the inferior quadrant of the vestibule is the coronary sinus. It runs a centimeter or so distant from the level of

the mitral valve hingeline (annulus) (Fig. 5.12) (see also Chapter 9). When the coronary sinus can be traced to the remnant of the oblique left atrial vein (ligament of Marshall), the remnant can be seen to run in the fold of atrial wall ("ridge," as described above) that lies between the left atrial appendage and the left superior pulmonary vein.

Left atrial appendage

Because the left atrium is situated posteriorly relative to the other cardiac chambers, only its appendage is visible when the heart is viewed from the front. The appendage forms the superior part of the left cardiac border (Fig. 5.13; see also Chapter 2).

Characteristically, the left appendage is a finger-like extension from the atrial chamber and it usually points anteriorly and superiorly, overlying the left ventricular wall. Its ostium (the orifice opening into the chamber) lies immediately above the level of the left atrioventricular groove. The circumflex branch of the left coronary artery runs close to the basal margin of the ostium (Fig. 5.14).

Usually the left phrenic nerve descends along the fibrous pericardium in close relation to the location of the appendage. As the appendage is within the confines of the pericardium, lying between the free wall of the left ventricle and the pericardial sac, its

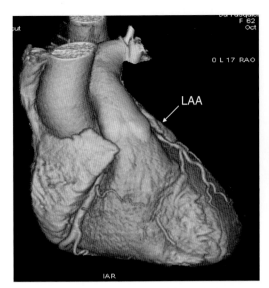

Figure 5.13   3D volume rendering of the entire heart from the anterior perspective. The left atrial appendage (LAA) forms the superior part of the left heart border.

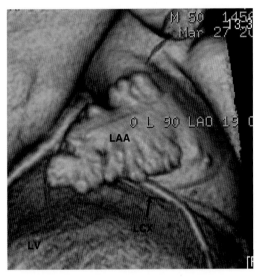

Figure 5.14   3D volume rendering of the left atrial appendage (LAA) and its relationships with surrounding structures. LV = left ventricle; LCX = left circumflex artery.

emptying and filling may be significantly affected by left ventricular function (Fig. 5.15).

Anatomically, the left appendage is likely the most variable structure of the entire heart. It may be a long, tubular, hooked structure with one, two, three or more lobes that spread in different directions (Fig. 5.16). It has a narrow junction with the

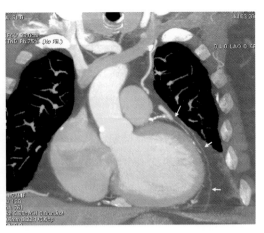

Figure 5.15   MIP projection coronal view. The arrows point to the course of the left phrenic nerve.

venous component of the atrium. Unlike the right side, the junction of the left appendage with its own atrium is not marked either externally or internally by a crest or groove (Fig. 5.17).

The pectinate muscles appear as interlacing fine ridges lining the lumen of the appendage. Without a terminal crest for anchorage, these ridges tend to be less regularly arranged than in the right appendage (Fig. 5.18).

Left ventricle

The morphological left ventricle forms the apex and the lower part of the left heart border. It is shaped like a cone (ellipsoid of revolution) with its long axis directed from the apex to the base (Figs. 5.19 and 5.20). Short-axis cross-sections, perpendicular to the long axis, reveal a roughly circular geometry (Fig. 5.21). The endocardial surface is irregular relative to the epicardial surface because of the two groups of papillary muscles and trabeculations (Fig. 5.22). Sections parallel to the ventricular long axis reveal an ellipsoid geometry. There are important variations in wall thickness, caused mainly by variation in the amount of circumferentially oriented mid-wall fibers (Fig. 5.23).

Stress develops when pressure is applied to a cross-sectional area. According to the Laplace law, wall stress in the left ventricle is determined by the intracavitary pressure × radius of curvature/ twice the wall thickness (Fig. 5.24). Because of the conical shape of the left ventricle, the end-diastolic

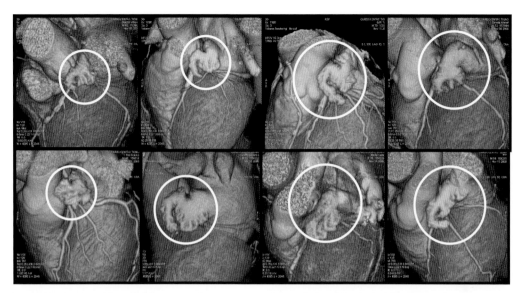

Figure 5.16 A composition of eight consecutive patients showing the extreme variability of the shape of the left atrial appendage (white circle). It may be long, tubular, or hooked with one, two, three or more lobes spreading in different directions.

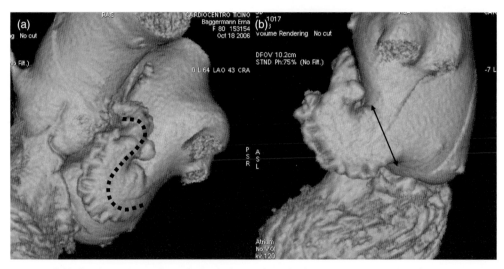

Figure 5.17 (a,b) The electronic cast shows the hooked structure of the left atrial appendage and its narrow junction with the venous component of the atrium (arrow). The junction between the left atrium and the left atrial appendage is not marked by any sulcus or crest.

circumferential radius of curvature gradually decreases from base to apex. Radius of curvature and wall thickness are related: wall thickness is smallest at the apex where the radius of curvature is also smallest. According to the Laplace law, the small radius of curvature compensates for the greater stress acting over the thinner apical wall (Fig. 5.25).

During systole the ventricle thickens radially (from the epicardium to the center of the cavity, in the direction of radii perpendicular to the long axis) (Fig. 5.26) and shortens from the base to apex along meridians (curved lines parallel to the long axis) (Fig. 5.27). Moreover, shortening also occurs circumferentially along curved lines in short-axis planes and, finally, the apex twists relative to the base (see also 3D Video clip 8, Left ventricle rotation ⊚). These simultaneous movements in different directions can be explained by the complex architecture of muscle fiber orientation. In the mid-wall (halfway between the epicardium and the endocardium) the fibers lie in the circumferential plane, aligned with the short-axis section. In the

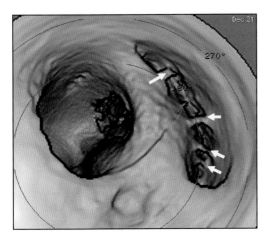

Figure 5.18 Virtual endoscopy of the left atrial appendage with its pectinate muscles (arrows).

subendocardium (approximately 10% of wall thickness from the endocardial surface), the fibers course upward and to the right averaging 60° oblique to the circumferential plane. Finally, in the subepicardium (10% of wall thickness closest to epicardial surface), the fibers course downward to the right averaging 60° oblique to the circumferential plane thus overlapping the subendocardial fibers at 120° (Fig. 5.28). The 3D electronic cast of left ventricle shows the helical disposition of the trabeculations. Whether this disposition is related to the subendocardial fibers is unknown (Fig. 5.29a,b).

Like the right ventricle, the left ventricle possesses an inlet, an apical trabecular component, and an outlet. The inlet component contains the mitral valve and extends from the atrioventricular junction to the attachment of the papillary muscles (Fig. 5.30a,b). The apical trabecular portion is the most characteristic feature of the morphological left ventricle and contains fine trabeculations (Fig. 5.31). This part helps identification because the left ventricle never possesses a septomarginal trabeculation or a moderator band.

In a sizable minority (in 40–50% of autopsy series) fibrous or fibromuscular bands (also known as false tendons) stretch across the left ventricle from the septum to the free wall. They can also tether to a papillary muscle, but unlike the chordae

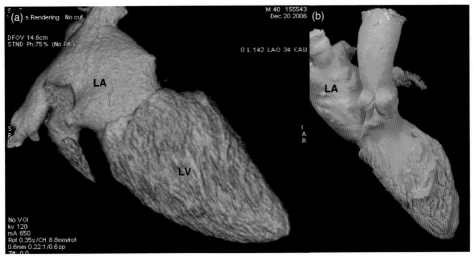

Figure 5.19 (a) "Electronic cast" showing the shape of the left ventricle. (b) Endocast preparation from a specimen in antero-posterior view. LA = left atrium; LV = left ventricle.

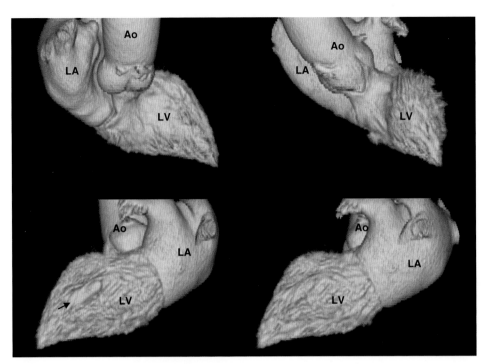

Figure 5.20 Electronic cast of the left ventricle (LV), left atrium (LA), and aorta (Ao) from different perspectives. The geometry of the left ventricle resembles an ellipsoid of revolution. The arrow marks the imprint of the anterior papillary muscle (see Video clip 5, Left ventricle).

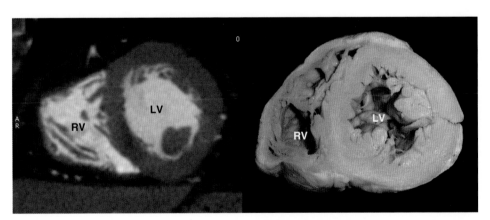

Figure 5.21 Short-axis cross-sectional slices and a specimen showing a roughly circular left ventricle with irregular endocardial surface. LV = left ventricle; RV = right ventricle.

tendineae, do not connect to the mitral leaflets. They are anatomic variants that should not be mistaken for abnormalities such as tumors, subaortic membranes, thrombus borders, and septal hypertrophy. Histological examination shows the false tendons to be composed of cardiac muscle, blood vessels, fibrous tissue, and Purkinje cells. False tendons might play a role in innocent murmurs or premature beats. Moreover, these fibromuscular bands may be involved as a part of the circuit in the genesis of ventricular tachycardia (Figs. 5.32a,b and 5.33).

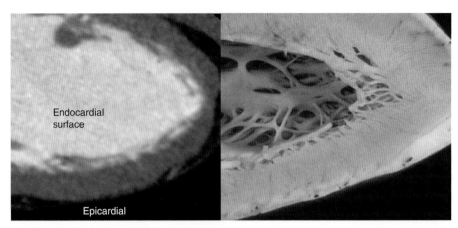

Figure 5.22   Magnified images of a portion of the left ventricular wall. The endocardial surface is more irregular than the epicardial surface because of the trabeculations.

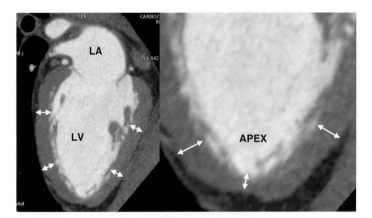

Figure 5.23   Long-axis slices showing the differences in wall thickness between anterior and inferior walls and the thin apex. LA = left atrium; LV = left ventricle.

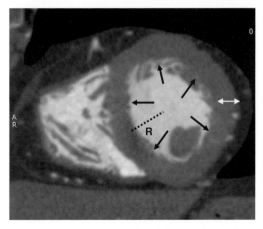

Figure 5.24   Short-axis view of the left ventricle showing the determinants of wall stress: the pressure inside the cavity (black arrows), the radius (dotted line), and the wall thickness (double white arrow). According to the Laplace law: stress = pressure × radius/twice the wall thickness.

The outlet component supports the aortic valve and consists of both muscular and fibrous portions. This is in contrast to the infundibulum of the right ventricle, which is comprised entirely of muscle. The septal portion of the left ventricular outflow tract, although primarily muscular, also includes the membranous portion of the ventricular septum (see Chapter 7). The posterior quadrant of the outflow tract consists of an extensive fibrous curtain that extends from the fibrous skeleton of the heart across the aortic leaflet of the mitral valve (Fig. 5.34), and supports the leaflets of the aortic valve in the area of aortic–mitral fibrous continuity (see Chapter 6). The lateral quadrant of the outflow tract is again muscular and consists of the lateral margin of the inner curvature of the heart.

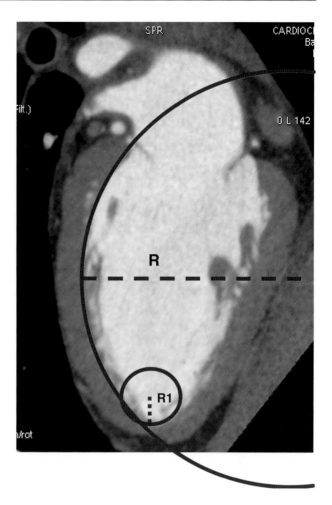

Figure 5.25   Long-axis slice of left ventricle. The radius of curvature of anterior wall (R) is greater than that of the apical wall (R1). According to the Laplace law, the small radius of curvature reduces the stress at the apex.

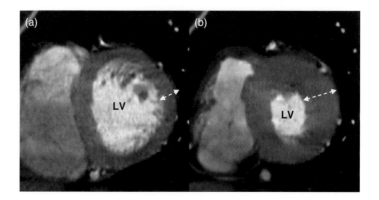

Figure 5.26   Short-axis view in diastole (a) and in systole (b) (see text and Video clip 6, Short axis function 👁). LV = left ventricle.

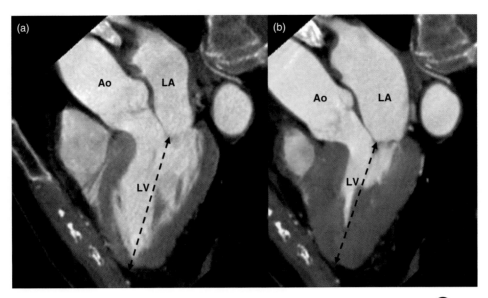

Figure 5.27   Long-axis view in diastole (a) and in systole (b) (see text and Video clip 7, Long axis function 👁). Ao = aorta; LA = left atrium; LV = left ventricle.

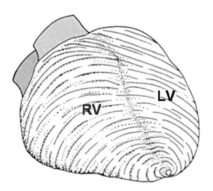

Subepicardial fibers (oblique)

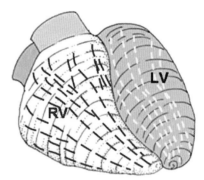

Mesocardial fibers (circumferential)
Subendocardial fibers (longitudinal)

Figure 5.28   The left ventricular wall has three major orientations of myofibers. The left-hand panel shows the oblique orientation in the subepicardium for both right and left ventricles (RV and LV). The right-hand panel shows the thick "layer" of circumferentially oriented myofibers in the mesocardium and the thin "layer" of myofibers in the subendocardium (broken lines).

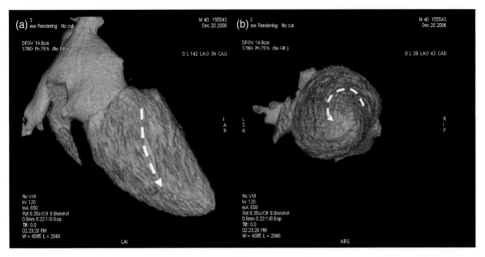

Figure 5.29   Electronic cast. (a) Anterior view showing the oblique course of trabeculations. (b) A view from the apex shows the helical disposition of the trabeculations.

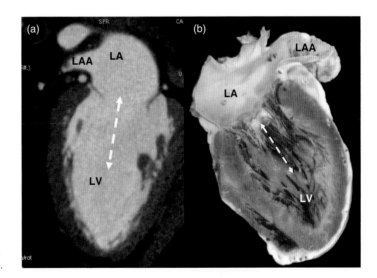

Figure 5.30   (a) Two-chamber-view slice, and (b) anatomic specimen showing the inlet part of the left ventricle extending from the atrioventricular junction to the attachment of papillary muscles (arrow). LV = left ventricle; LA = left atrium; LAA = left atrial appendage.

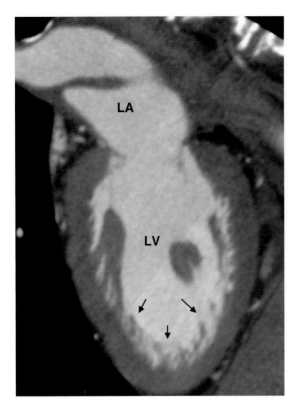

Figure 5.31 Two-chamber-view slice showing the fine trabeculations of the left ventricle. LA = left atrium; LV = left ventricle.

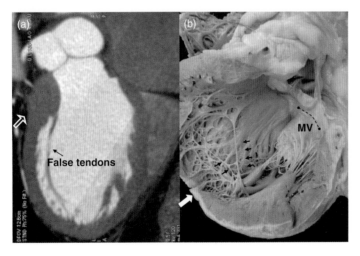

Figure 5.32 (a) Long-axis-view slice showing a false tendon running from the septum to the apex. (b) Anatomic specimen. The left ventricle is splayed open to show several false tendons (arrows) crossing the cavity of the left ventricle. Note the area of fibrous continuity between the aortic and the mitral valves (MV) (broken line) and the very thin muscular wall at the apex (white arrow).

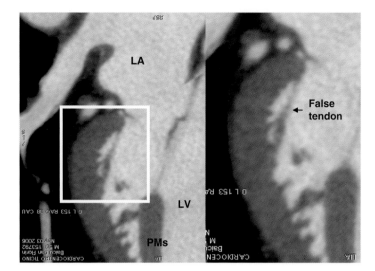

Figure 5.33 False tendon in the posterior wall. LA = left atrium; LV = left ventricle; PMs = papillary muscle.

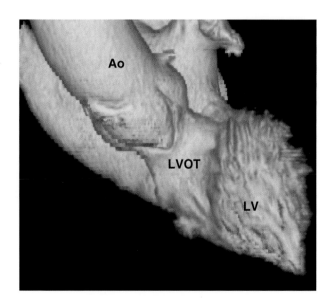

Figure 5.34 Electronic cast (left anterior oblique view) showing the left ventricular outflow tract cavity (LVOT). Ao = aorta; LV = left ventricle.

Suggested reading

Becker AE. Left atrial isthmus: anatomic aspects relevant for linear catheter ablation procedures in humans. *J Cardiovasc Electrophysiol* 2004;15:809–812.

Buckberg GD, Castella M, Gharib M, Saleh S. Structure/function interface with sequential shortening of basal and apical components of the myocardial band. *Eur J Cardiothorac Surg* 2006;29(Suppl 1):S75–S97.

Cirillo S, Bonamini R, Gaita F *et al*. Magnetic resonance angiography virtual endoscopy in the assessment of pulmonary veins before radiofrequency ablation procedures for atrial fibrillation. *Eur Radiol* 2004;14:2053–2060.

Ernst G, Stollberger C, Abzieher F *et al*. Morphology of the left atrial appendage. *Anat Rec* 1995;242:553–561.

Greenbaum RA, Ho SY, Gibson DG, Becker AE, Anderson RH. Left ventricular fibre architecture in man. *Br Heart J* 1981;45:248–263.

Ho SY, Sanchez-Quintana D, Cabrera JA, Anderson RH. Anatomy of the left atrium: implications for radiofrequency ablation of atrial fibrillation. *J Cardiovasc Electrophysiol* 1999;10:1525–1533.

Kato R, Lickfett L, Meininger G *et al*. Pulmonary vein anatomy in patients undergoing catheter ablation of atrial fibrillation: lessons learned by use of magnetic resonance imaging. *Circulation* 2003;107:2004–2010.

Le Grice IJ, Takayama Y, Covell JW. Transverse shear along myocardial cleavage planes provides a mechanism for normal systolic wall thickening. *Circ Res* 1995;77:182–193.

Lorenz CH, Pastorek JS, Bundy JM. Delineation of normal human left ventricular twist throughout systole by tagged cine magnetic resonance imaging. *J Cardiovasc Magn Reson* 2000;2:97–108.

McCulloch AD, Omens JH. Myocyte shearing, myocardial sheets, and microtubules. *Circ Res* 2006;98:1–3.

Rademakers FE, Rogers WJ, Guier WH *et al*. Relation of regional cross-fiber shortening to wall thickening in the intact heart. Three dimensional strain analysis by NMR tagging. *Circulation* 1994;89:1174–1182.

Sanchez-Quintana D, Cabrera JA, Climent V, Farre J, Weiglein A, Ho SY. How close are the phrenic nerves to cardiac structures? Implications for cardiac interventionalists. *J Cardiovasc Electrophysiol* 2005;16:309–313.

Sanchez-Quintana D, Garcia-Martinez V, Climent V, Hurle JM. Morphological changes in the normal pattern of ventricular myoarchitecture in the developing human heart. *Anat Rec* 1995;243:483–495.

Schwartzman D, Lacomis J, Wigginton WG. Characterization of left atrium and distal pulmonary vein morphology using multidimensional computed tomography. *J Am Coll Cardiol* 2003;41:1349–1357.

CHAPTER 6

The Cardiac Valves

Aortic valve

Aortic root

The aortic root may be defined as the portion of the left ventricular outflow tract that supports the leaflets of the aortic valve, delineated by the sinutubular ridge superiorly and the bases of the valve leaflets inferiorly. It comprises the aortic valve leaflets and their hingelines, the sinuses, the interleaflet triangles, the ventriculo-arterial junction, and the sinutubular junction. These components all work in concert to accomplish the role of the aortic root, which is to allow unimpeded forward flow when open and prevention of backflow when closed. Like the mitral valve apparatus, the complex interactions of all the components of the aortic root are both its strength and its potential weakness. Disruption of any component by disease processes such as aortic annuloectasia affects all the other components and can alter the biomechanics of the whole system. The aortic root is centrally located in the heart. Seen in profile, it lies behind the subpulmonary muscular infundibulum and anterior to the atria (Fig. 6.1). Because of its central location, the aortic valve is related to each of the cardiac chambers and cardiac valves (Fig. 6.2).

The annulus (ring hingeline)

Similar to the pulmonary valve, the semilunar hingelines of the aortic leaflets give a crown-shaped appearance to the fibrous thickening that forms the so-called annulus. It is a condensation of collagenous tissue that follows the semilunar contour

Anatomy of the Heart by Multislice Computed Tomography.
By Francesco Fulvio Faletra, Natesa G. Pandian and Siew Yen Ho. Published 2008 by Wiley-Blackwell Publishing, ISBN: 978-1-4051-8055-9.

of the valvar attachment. As with the pulmonary valve, the semilunar attachment extends across the ventriculo-arterial junction. Importantly, the "annulus" is not shaped like a conventional ring. The summits are at the commissures, which are the highest points of the valvar closure lines. They reach to the level of the sinutubular junction whereas the nadirs cross into ventricular tissues. This arrangement gives the valve the flexibility that would not be possible if the ring was a circular band (Figs. 6.3 and 6.4).

Aortic leaflets

The normal aortic valve has three semilunar leaflets. The leaflets seldom are perfectly equal in size. Each leaflet has a semicircular hingeline, a body, and a coapting surface (Fig. 6.5).

The three leaflets meet centrally along zones of apposition where adjacent leaflets coapt (Fig. 6.6). At the center of each zone is a thickened nodule, called the nodule of Arantius. Peripherally, adjacent to the commissures, the surfaces of coaptation are thinner and may contain small perforations in normal valves. These perforations have no hemodynamic impact because they occur on or above (distal to) the zones of apposition.

During systole, the leaflets are pushed aside, away from the center of the aortic lumen and into the sinuses, whereas during diastole they fall back passively to obliterate the lumen. The curvilinear attachment between the aortic valve leaflets and aortic root wall allows for stress sharing. This arrangement enables the high stresses carried by each leaflet during closure to be shared with the aortic root wall (Fig. 6.7).

The sinuses of Valsalva

Behind each leaflet, the aortic wall bulges outward to form the sinus of Valsalva. The sinuses of

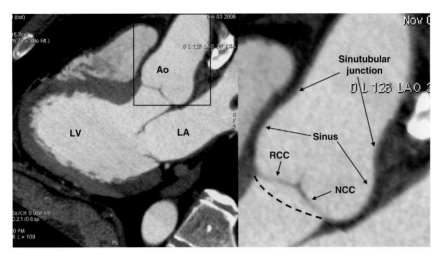

Figure 6.1 The aortic valve apparatus is composed of several components: the leaflets, the sinuses of Valsalva, the sinutubular junction, the ventriculo-arterial junction (black dotted line), and the interleaflet triangles (not seen in this figure). Note the location of the aortic valve behind the right ventricular outflow tract (RVOT) and in front of the transverse pericardial sinus (*).
Ao = aorta; LV = left ventricle; LA = left atrium; RC = right coronary leaflet; NC = non-coronary leaflet.

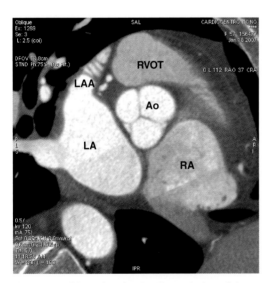

Figure 6.2 Oblique slice showing short-axis view of the heart at its base. Image shows the aorta (Ao), the left atrium (LA), the left atrial appendage (LAA) and the right ventricular outflow tract (RVOT). The aortic valve is located to the right and posterior to RVOT and forms the centerpiece of the heart. RA = right atrium.

Valsalva occupy the greater part of the aortic root. The sinuses are composed primarily of elastic tissue, and they contain the orifices (ostia) of the coronary arteries. In cross-section, the aortic root at this level is trilobed. The trilobed configuration reduces the radius of curvature of the aortic root thus minimizing the diastolic stress against the aortic wall (Fig. 6.8). As first recognized by Leonardo Da Vinci, the sinuses lead to the creation of eddies within the flowing blood during ventricular ejection. This eddy formation assists in two functions: one is valve closure, and the other is aiding or ensuring coronary ostial perfusion. Two of the three aortic sinuses give rise to coronary arteries, hence their designations as right, left and non-coronary sinuses. The latter is usually the largest.

The sinutubular junction is a ridge of aortic wall that is thicker than the adjacent sinuses. It forms a circle joining the peaks of the commissures. It delineates the beginning of the tubular ascending aorta (Fig. 6.9).

The interleaflet triangles

Because of the semilunar attachment of the aortic leaflets, there are three interleaflet triangles that are extensions of the left ventricular outflow tract because they are located beneath the level of the leaflets when the valve is in the closed position. The apex of each triangle reaches near to the sinutubular junction where the attachments of adjacent leaflets meet together forming the "commissures" (Fig. 6.10).

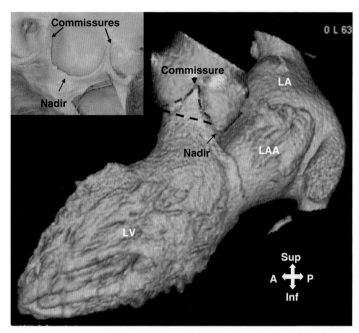

Figure 6.3 3D electronic cast of the left ventricle (LV) and the left atrium (LA) with the aortic root colored in pink and the left ventricle in purple. The semilunar attachments (red dashed line) of the valvar leaflets are arranged in crown-like fashion (see inset of anatomic specimen). The black dashed line marks the ventriculo-arterial junction. Inset: anatomic specimen showing the crown-shaped appearance of the cusps' attachment. LAA = left atrial appendage.

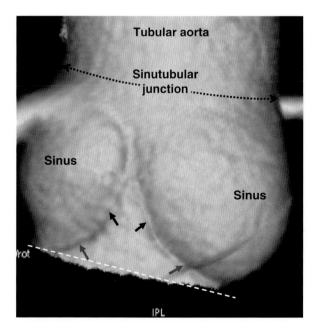

Figure 6.4 3D volume rendering external view of the aortic root. The sinutubular junction distinguishes the tubular portion of the aorta from the sinuses. The arrows point to the condensations of collagenous tissue ("annulus" or hingeline) where the leaflets attach in semilunar (crown-shaped) fashion to the aortic root. The dotted line represents the level of the ventriculo-arterial junction that passes through the hingelines. Anatomically, the lower parts of the sinuses delimited by hingelines (blue arrows) are composed of ventricular tissues. Thus, the right coronary and part of the left coronary sinuses contain ventricular myocardium, a relevant feature for electrophysiologists ablating foci of idiopathic ventricular tachycardia.

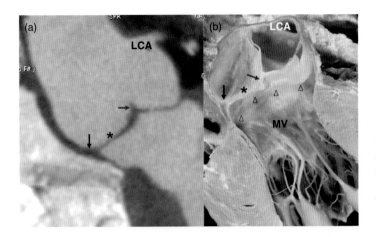

Figure 6.5 (a) Oblique slice and (b) the corresponding anatomic specimen. Each leaflet has a hinge point (black arrow), a body (*), and a coapting surface (red arrow). LCA = left coronary artery; MV = mitral valve.

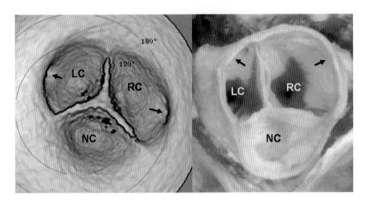

Figure 6.6 3D virtual endoscopic view of aortic leaflets in closed position and a similar display of a heart specimen viewed from the ascending aorta. The arrows indicate the orifices leading to the left and right coronary arteries. LC = left coronary; RC = right coronary; NC = non-coronary leaflet.

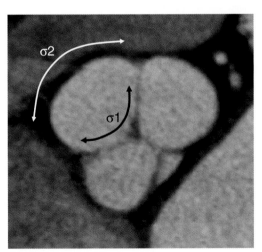

Figure 6.7 Scheme of stress (σ) in leaflets and wall of the aortic root. Because the leaflets are thinner than the wall, the leaflet stresses ($\sigma1$) are higher than the root wall stresses ($\sigma2$). However, the curvilinear attachment at the sinuses enables the high leaflet stress to be partially transferred to the root wall, thereby decreasing the stress on the leaflets.

The triangle between the right coronary and non-coronary aortic sinuses incorporates within it the membranous part of the septum (Fig. 6.11). The latter is a landmark for the course of the atrioventricular bundle of the cardiac conduction system. The triangle between the left coronary and the non-coronary aortic sinuses forms part of the aortic-mitral valvar curtain (Fig. 6.12). The inter-leaflet triangles, therefore, are exposed to ventricular hemodynamics.

The ventriculo-arterial junction
Toward the proximal end of the aortic root is the anatomic ventriculo-arterial junction. This is unequivocally circular in shape, and is below the level of origin of the coronary arteries. It is at the ventriculo-arterial junction that surgeons sew prosthetic valves, taking particular care in the region of the membranous septum. The junction crosses the semilunar hingelines, resulting in

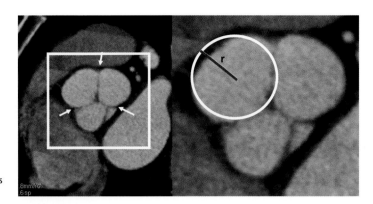

Figure 6.8 The trilobate configuration reduces the radius of curvature, thus minimizing the stress upon the sinuses.

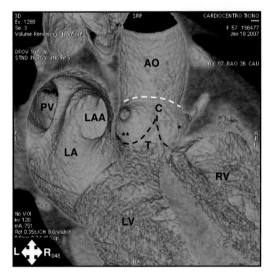

Figure 6.9 3D endocardial surface modality looking from the back of the heart toward the front, depicting the crown-shaped (black dotted line) insertions of the left (**) and right (*) aortic leaflets with the commissure (C) between. The anterior interleaflet triangle (T) adjoins muscular ventricular septum. The dotted white line marks the sinutubular junction. The orifices of the left and right coronary arteries are also visible (arrows). AO = aorta; LA = left atrium; PV = pulmonary vein; LV = left ventricle; RV = right ventricle.

basal ring (Fig. 6.13). This level corresponds to the echocardiographic "annulus" when measurements of the diameter of the aortic valve are made.

Mitral valve

The mitral valve apparatus comprises annulus, valvar leaflets, tendinous cords that attach to the leaflets, and papillary muscles that anchor the cords. Also important for its functioning is the left atrial musculature inserting to the leaflets at the annulus and the ventricular myocardium to which the papillary muscles are attached. The normal mitral valve has two leaflets that, conventionally, are described as anterior and posterior leaflets. With tomographic imaging of the heart *in situ*, it is obvious that these leaflets are not in anterior or posterior positions. But because surgeons continue to use this convention, we will continue to use the term "anterior" for the leaflet that is nearest to the aortic valve and "posterior" for the mural leaflet. Similarly, the "commissures" (ends of the zone of apposition between leaflets), and the papillary muscles are referred to as antero-lateral and postero-medial.

Mitral annulus
The mitral annulus has an elliptical or D-shaped configuration (Fig. 6.14). The straight border accommodates the aortic valve allowing the latter to be wedged between the ventricular septum and the mitral valve (Fig. 6.15a). In this region, the aortic valve is in fibrous continuity with the anterior leaflet of the mitral valve (mitral-aortic continuity or mitral-aortic curtain). Expansions

small segments of ventricular myocardium being enclosed within the right sinus and part of the left sinus of the aortic root. The non-coronary sinus has no muscular incorporation because it adjoins the aortic-mitral curtain (Figs. 6.10–6.12).

The basal ring
An imaginary line joining the nadirs of the semilunar hingelines forms a circle, described as the

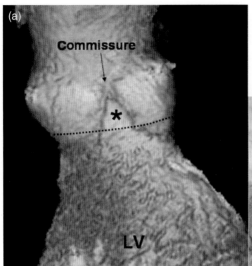

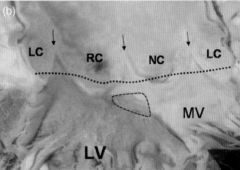

Figure 6.10 (a) 3D volume rendering reconstruction of aortic root, external view, to show the interleaflet triangle (*) between the semilunar attachments of the leaflets. (b) A heart specimen opened longitudinally through the left coronary (LC) sinus of the aortic valve. The leaflets have been removed to show the accretions of fibrous tissue that make up the hingelines that approximate at the commissures (arrows). Note the ventriculo-arterial junction intersects the semilunar hingelines. The nadirs of the right (RC) and left (LC) sinuses contain ventricular myocardium whereas the non-coronary (NC) sinus and part of the left sinus have no ventricular muscle because they are in fibrous continuity with the mitral valve. The interleaflet triangle between the right (RC) and non-coronary (NC) sinuses abuts the membranous septum (encircled by a red broken line), which is in proximity to the atrioventricular conduction bundle. Anatomically, the interleaflet fibrous triangles are arterial and lead outside the heart. Hemodynamically, however, they are ventricular because they occupy the ventricular side of the valve when the leaflets are in the closed position. LV = left ventricle; MV = mitral valve.

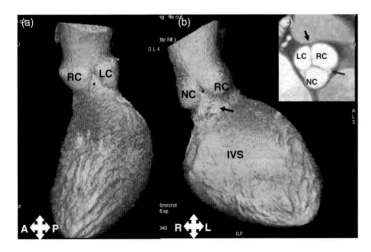

Figure 6.11 (a) 3D volume rendering reconstruction of the interleaflet triangle (*) between the right coronary (RC) and the left coronary (LC) sinuses. (b) The interleaflet triangle (*) between the non-coronary (NC) and the right coronary (RC) sinuses. The arrow marks the membranous septum. (c) Oblique slice showing the interleaflet triangles.

of fibrous tissues at either extreme of the area of continuity form the rigid right and left fibrous trigones (Fig. 6.15b–d). The maximum stress on the mitral valve is at the trigones (Fig. 6.16). The clinical implication is that all annuloplasties must be anchored to the trigones for firm support. The annulus does not lie in a single plane but has a saddle-shaped configuration. There is a "peak" in the midpoint of the anterior segment of the annulus and another "peak" in the midpoint of the posterior segment whereas the "valleys" lie near the commissures (Fig. 6.17). The anterior "peak" rises higher than

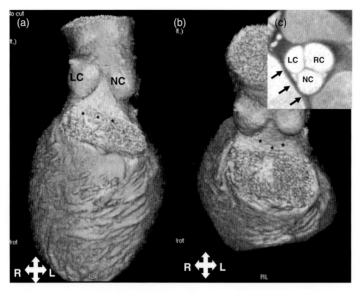

Figure 6.12 (a,b) 3D volume rendering reconstruction of the interleaflet triangle between the left coronary sinus (LC) and the non-coronary sinus (NC) showing the fibrous continuity with the mitral valve (***). (c) Oblique view showing the mitro-aortic continuity. RC = right coronary sinus.

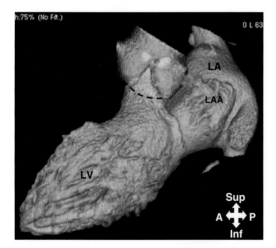

Figure 6.13 3D electronic cast of the left ventricle and the left atrium with the aortic root colored in pink and the left ventricle in purple. The black dashed line marks the basal ring. LV = left ventricle; LA = left atrium; LAA = left atrial appendage.

the posterior "peak." The configuration and size of the annulus vary constantly during the cardiac cycle. This hyperbolic paraboloid shape reduces significantly the mechanical stress. It is this knowledge that motivated the development of flexible rings for mitral annuloplasty.

Leaflets

The leaflets are the most important components of the mitral apparatus for competent valve closure. They meet at the closure line forming a single zone of apposition (Fig. 6.18). The "commissures" are the extreme ends of the zone of apposition. The commissures do not reach the annulus, but end about 5 mm short. Thus from a strictly anatomic point of view, being hinged along the entire annular circumference, the mitral leaflets can be considered as a single veil with the anterior leaflet hanging like a curtain between the left ventricular inflow and outflow tracts (Fig. 6.19). The hingeline of the anterior leaflet occupies one-third of the annular circumference (nearly 3 cm). Being roughly triangular in shape, the anterior leaflet is deeper than the posterior leaflet (Figs. 6.19 and 6.20). The latter is long and narrow and is attached to the two-thirds of the remaining annular circumference. Thus, the overall orifice areas covered by each leaflet are equivalent. Small identations, termed clefts, usually divide the posterior leaflets into three scallops (Figs. 6.18 and 6.21) but quite often there are four or more scallops. Using the surgeon's terminology, these scallops are denoted from lateral to medial as P1, P2 and P3 (P stands for posterior), arbitrarily apportioning the leaflet into thirds. The corresponding areas of the anterior leaflet are denoted A1, A2

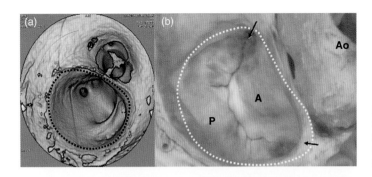

Figure 6.14 (a) Virtual endoscopy and (b) anatomic specimen both showing the "D-shaped" annulus configuration (dotted line). P = posterior; A = anterior.

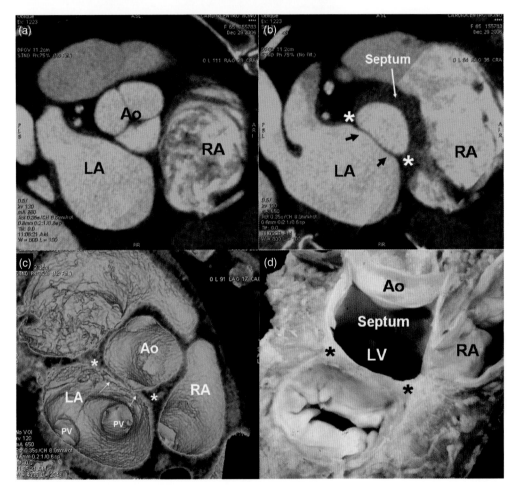

Figure 6.15 (a,b) Axial slices at different levels, (c) 3D endocardial surface modality and (d) anatomic specimen showing the fibrous continuity between aortic and mitral valves. * = trigone; Ao = aorta; RA = right atrium; LA = left atrium; LV = left ventricle; PV = pulmonary vein.

and A3, although any anatomic indentations can be observed (Fig. 6.18). In the normal valve, the total leaflet area is approximately twice that of the mitral orifice. This tissue abundance may account for the success of mitral repair compared with aortic valve repair, where lack of available tissue is a constant limitation. In both leaflets two different zones can be distinguished – a clear and a rough zone. This distinction is more evident in the anterior leaflet. The tendinous cords mainly insert

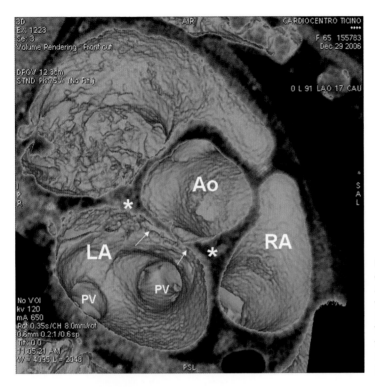

Figure 6.16 Magnified image of panel (c) of Fig. 6.15 showing an endocardial view from the ventricular perspective. Arrows indicate the mitro-aortic curtain. The two asterisks indicate the trigones. Ao = aorta; RA = right atrium; LA = left atrium; PV = pulmonary vein.

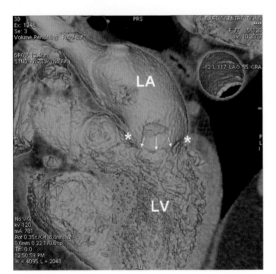

Figure 6.17 3D long-axis endocardial surface modality. Peaks are located in the mid-points of the anterior and posterior segments (*) whereas "valleys" lie near the commissures (arrows). LA = left atrium; LV = left ventricle.

to the ventricular side of the rough zone making the latter appear irregular and thicker than the clear zone. In systole, the atrial sides of both rough zones meet each other to ensure valvar competence along the closure line. The surface of leaflet coaptation is 5–8 mm deep along the zone of apposition allowing the valve to accommodate a moderate degree of annular dilation without becoming incompetent. The clear zone, particularly visible in the anterior leaflet, is thin and translucent. In systole, the clear zone of the anterior leaflet bulges toward the anterior cavity (Fig. 6.23).

Tendinous cords (chordae tendineae)

These cords are fibrous string-like structures on the ventricular surfaces of the leaflets. The majority connect the rough zone and the free edges of leaflets to papillary muscles. Unlike the tricuspid valve, the normal mitral valve does not have cords attaching the leaflets to the ventricular septum. Because cords usually branch several times distal to their origin, there are four or five times more cords attached to the leaflets than to the papillary muscles. There is a wide variability from heart to heart in cordal arrangement and only a general organization can be recognized. One of the more useful classifications distinguishes tendinous cords into first-, second- and third-order cords according to their insertion onto

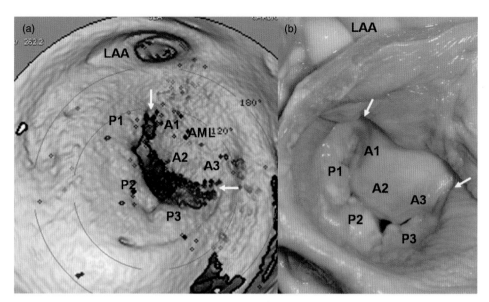

Figure 6.18 Virtual endoscopy (a) and anatomic specimen (b) from an atrial perspective. Two main identations divide the mitral veil in the anterior mitral leaflet (AML) and the posterior leaflets (arrows). Posterior leaflets are subdivided in three scallops (P1, P2 and P3). A1, A2 and A3 are the corresponding regions of the anterior leaflet. LAA = left atrial appendage.

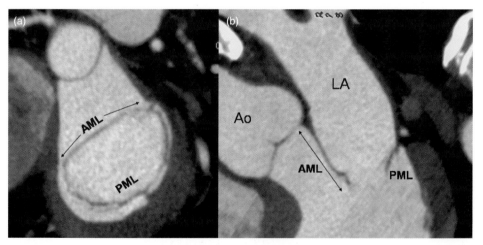

Figure 6.19 Oblique slices. The anterior mitral leaflet (AML) occupies one-third of the annular circumference (a), but is deeper than the posterior mitral leaflets (PML). (b) The overall orifice areas covered by each leaflet are therefore equivalent Ao = aorta; LA = left atrium.

the leaflet's margin, rough zone or basal areas, respectively. The first-order cords are thought to prevent valvar incompetence; the second-order cords, which include some of the thickest cords (known as strut cords), maintain mitral–papillary muscle–ventricle wall continuity, thus supporting longitudinal left ventricle shortening and left ventricular function (Fig. 6.24). The role of the basal cords, which connect the basal area of the posterior leaflet directly to the ventricular wall, is not clear.

At each "commissure" is a distinctive cord (commissural cord) that branches into a fan-shape to insert into the adjacent leaflets. The "fan" is open when the leaflets move apart and it closes when the leaflets come together.

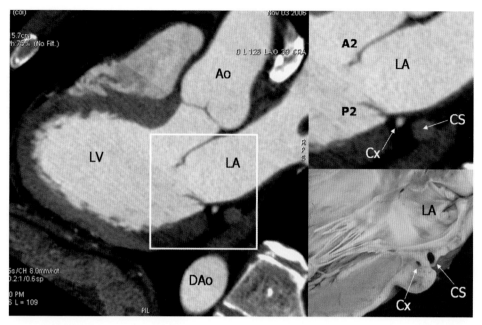

Figure 6.20 Oblique slice showing long-axis view of the left ventricle. Magnified image in the upper right corner and the corresponding anatomic specimen in the lower right corner showing mitral leaflets (A2 and P2), left circumflex artery (Cx) and coronary sinus (CS). Descending aorta (DAo) in the short axis is also displayed in the main panel. LV = left ventricle; LA = left atrium; Ao = aorta.

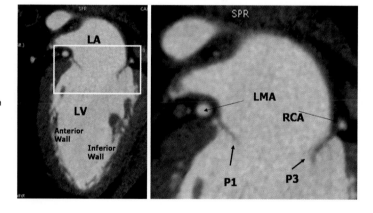

Figure 6.21 Oblique slice showing a two-chamber view in diastole. The lateral (P1) and medial (P3) scallops are shown in the magnified image. Note the left main artery (LMA) and the right coronary artery (RCA) in short-axis view. LA = left atrium; LV = left ventricle.

Papillary muscles

The papillary muscles are considered as a left ventricular muscular protuberance that anchors the cords to the left ventricular wall. Rupture of one of their heads results in severe valvar regurgitation. Viewed from the atrial aspect, the two groups are located beneath the commissures, occupying antero-lateral and postero-medial positions (Figs. 6.25 and 6.26). The arrangement of the papillary muscles in two groups allows the mitral valve to be distinguished from the tricuspid valve. Generally larger than the posteromedial muscle, the anterolateral papillary muscle is supplied by an artery derived from the circumflex or anterior descending branch of the left coronary artery (Fig. 6.27). Because most people have right dominance of the coronary pattern (see Chapter 8), it is the right coronary artery that most often supplies the postero-medial papillary muscle (Fig. 6.28). Papillary muscles are conceptualized as being

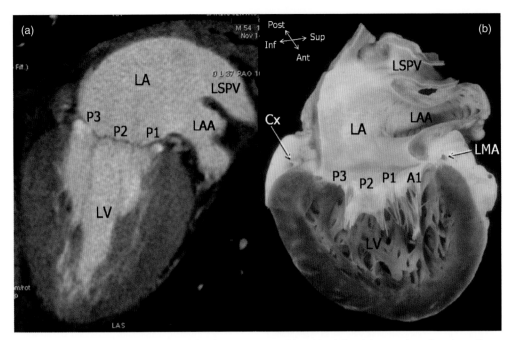

Figure 6.22   (a) Oblique slice showing a two-chamber view in systole. (b) The corresponding anatomic specimen. The three scallops, P1, P2 and P3, of the posterior leaflets are shown. LA = left atrium; LV = left ventricle; LAA = left atrial appendage; Cx = circumflex artery; LMA = left main artery; LSPV = left superior pulmonary vein.

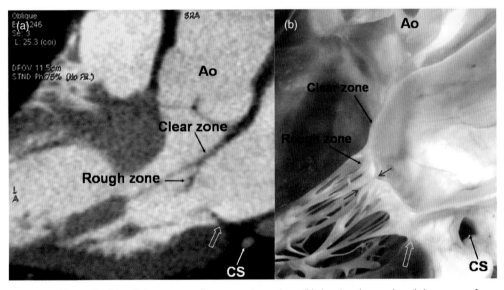

Figure 6.23   Oblique slice (a) and the corresponding anatomic specimen (b) showing the rough and clear zones of the anterior mitral leaflet. Ao = aorta; CS = coronary sinus.

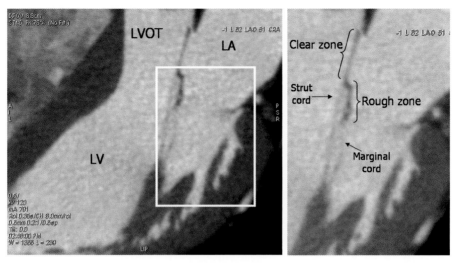

Figure 6.24 Oblique slice. In the magnified image (right) strut and marginal chordae as well as the clear and rough zones can also be distinguished. LA = left atrium; LV = left ventricle; LVOT = left ventricular outflow track.

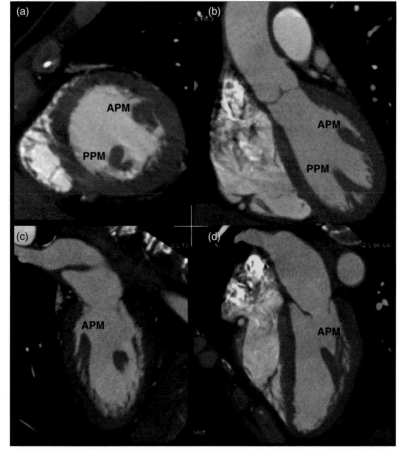

Figure 6.25 (a) Short-axis view, (b) coronal plane, (c) two-chamber and (d) four-chamber view showing anterior (APM) and posterior (PPM) papillary muscles.

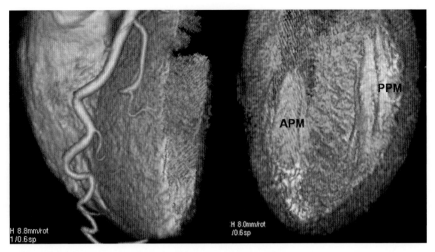

Figure 6.26   3D volume rendering image cropped in long-axis orientation. The lateral wall and the contrast have been "electronically" removed. Both anterior (APM) and posterior (PPM) papillary muscles are shown in 3D volume rendering format.

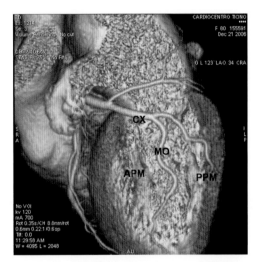

Figure 6.27   3D volume rendering. Image was cropped to visualize both papillary muscles. The coronary vessels were superimposed to show the relationships between circumflex coronary artery (CX), marginal branch (MO) and anterior papillary muscle (APM). PPM = posterior papillary muscle.

directly continuous with the solid portion of the heart wall, the compact myocardium, but tomographic imaging has consistently shown that the bases of the papillary muscles are not solid. Instead, they are composed of muscular continuations from the trabeculations that line the ventricular cavity (Figs. 6.29 and 6.30).

Tricuspid valve

Just like the mitral valve, the tricuspid valve guards the junction between atrium and ventricle and is also described as an atrioventricular valve. Its apparatus comprises "annulus" or hingeline, leaflets, tendinous cords and papillary muscles.

Tricuspid annulus
The tricuspid valve has an "annulus" to which the leaflets are hinged. Although "annulus" implies a well-formed collagenous ring, this is far from the case in the tricuspid valve. Collagenous accretions are seldom found. The hingeline has an elliptical shape that nearly mirrors the mitral "annulus" with straight septal and curved mural components (Fig. 6.31a). Moreover, recent studies have demonstrated a saddle-shaped configuration of the tricuspid "annulus" with the peaks in anterior and posterior positions, and the valley between medial and lateral positions (Fig. 6.31b).

Leaflets
Generally the valve has three leaflets – the medial or septal, the antero-superior and the posterior or inferior leaflets (Figs. 6.32 and 6.33). Attitudinally, antero-superior and inferior describe the locations better than anterior and posterior. Fan-shaped commissural cords support the peripheral ends of the zones of coaptation between adjacent leaflets. The commissures are designated antero-septal,

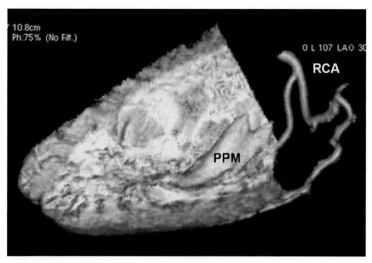

Figure 6.28   3D volume rendering. The heart was "electronically" dissected to show the relationship between the right coronary artery (RCA) and the posterior papillary muscle (PPM).

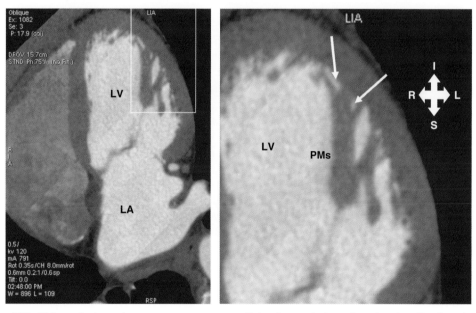

Figure 6.29   Oblique slice in up-down "echocardiographic" format. The base of the papillary muscle (PMs) joins with the network of trabeculae carneae lining the ventricular cavity rather than directly to the solid portion of the heart wall. LA = left atrium; LV = left ventricle.

antero-inferior and inferior. In some hearts, the divisions between leaflets are not so clear and some leaflets may have further subdivisions into scallops. In others, the division between antero-superior and inferior leaflets is not clear so some surgeons consider these as a unique leaflet with several scallops and call it the mural leaflet.

The septal leaflet (Fig. 6.34) has some characteristic features. First, it has multiple tendinous cords attaching it directly to the ventricular septum (Fig. 6.35). Second, its hinge is attached closer to the apex than that of the mitral leaflet. The difference in levels of attachment between the two atrioventricular valves, an offset arrangement, places

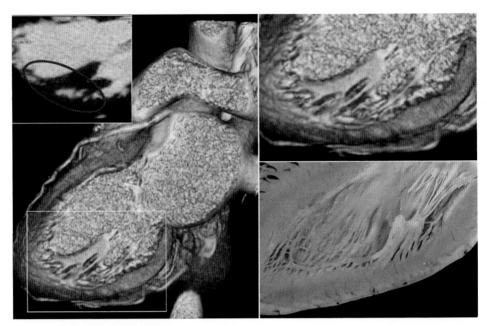

Figure 6.30 3D volume rendering images cropped in long-axis orientation. Magnified image of oblique slice in the left upper corner; magnified image of 3D volume rendering in the right upper corner and the corresponding anatomic specimen in the right lower corner showing the same papillary muscle insertion architecture.

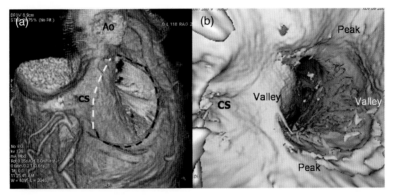

Figure 6.31 (a) 3D volume rendering format. Perspective from above and behind after removing the right atrium. The elliptical shape of tricuspid annulus with straight septal (dashed white line) and curved mural (dashed black line) components. (b) 3D virtual endoscopy. Tricuspid "annulus" has a saddle-shaped configuration with the peak in superior and inferior positions and the valley in medial and lateral positions. Ao = aorta; CS = ostium of coronary sinus.

part of the muscular ventricular septum in an atrioventricular position, and this is evident when cutting the heart just behind the aortic root in a four-chamber slice (Fig. 6.36). Although previously described as the muscular atrioventricular septum, closer examination has shown that it is not strictly septal. Instead, it has a sandwich-like arrangement of right atrial wall and ventricular septum with epicardial fat between. A slice tilted slightly more cephalad will show the hingeline of the septal leaflet bisecting the membranous septum into atrioventricular and interventricular components on the right heart aspect (Fig. 6.37); the aortic root is also revealed on this cut.

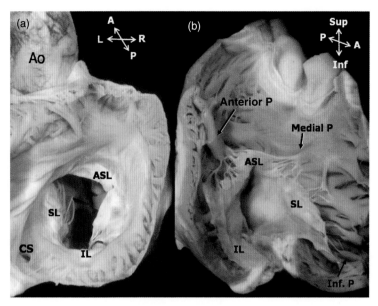

Figure 6.32 The tricuspid orifice viewed from (a) the atrial aspect and (b) the ventricular aspect to show the antero-superior (ASL), inferior (IL) and septal (SL) leaflets and commissures supported by the respective papillary muscles (P). Ao = aorta; CS = coronary sinus.

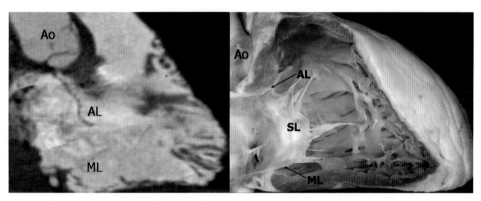

Figure 6.33 Oblique slice and comparable view of heart specimen. Antero-superior (AL), inferior or mural (ML) and septal (SL) leaflets are partially visible. Ao = aorta.

Papillary muscles

The arrangement of the papillary muscles supporting the tricuspid valve is more varied than that for the mitral valve. Usually, the antero-superior leaflet is supported by a large papillary muscle that arises from the moderator band (see also Chapter 4) (Fig. 6.38). Sometimes the muscle has two heads (Fig. 6.39). It is common to find cords from the antero-superior papillary muscle inserting to the mid-portion of the leaflet as well as to the antero-inferior commissure. By contrast, the antero-septal commissure is supported by a small papillary muscle, the medial papillary muscle, which inserts to the septomarginal trabeculation on the ventricular septum (Fig. 6.40). In some hearts, the medial papillary muscle is poorly formed whereas in others it is represented by a cluster of minute papillary muscles. The inferior leaflet is supported by several small papillary muscles that arise from the diaphragmatic wall of the right ventricle

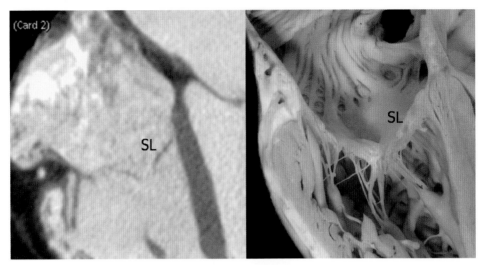

Figure 6.34 Oblique slice and comparable cut of heart specimen. The septal leaflet (SL) is hinged to the septum.

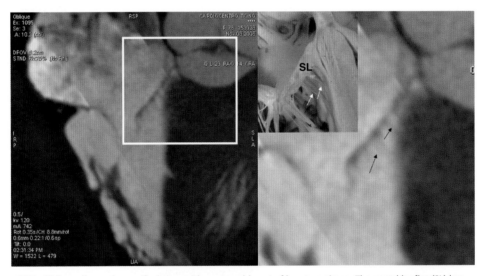

Figure 6.35 Oblique slice and magnified view with comparable cut of heart specimen. The septal leaflet (SL) has multiple tendinous cords (arrows) attaching it directly to the ventricular septum.

(Fig. 6.41). Often they are very small and appear as no more than small branches of cords arising directly from the wall. The septal leaflet is characterized by having cordal attachments directly to the septum (Fig. 6.35).

Pulmonary valve

The pulmonary valve is virtually identical in design to the aortic valve with the exception that the semilunar pulmonary leaflets are slightly thinner than the aortic leaflets and the sinuses are less prominent. Its location is anterior, superior and slightly to the left of the aortic valve (Figs. 6.42–6.44). Usually two of the three sinuses of the pulmonary valve "face" the right and left coronary sinuses of the aortic valve although the "facing" may be slightly offset in some cases. The right ventricular outlet is a muscular funnel termed the subpulmonary infundibulum. It supports the pulmonary valve

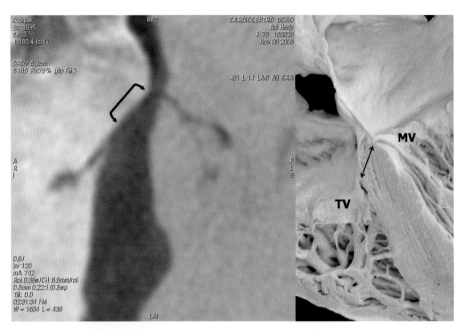

Figure 6.36 Oblique slice and heart specimen showing the hinge of the septal leaflet toward the cardiac crux. The offset between tricuspid and mitral hingelines results in the crest of the muscular ventricular septum being located between the right atrium and the left ventricle (double-headed arrow). This part of the heart gives a sandwich arrangement of right atrial myocardium overlying epicardial fat from the crux, which in turn overlies the ventricular septum.
MV = mitral valve; TV = tricuspid valve.

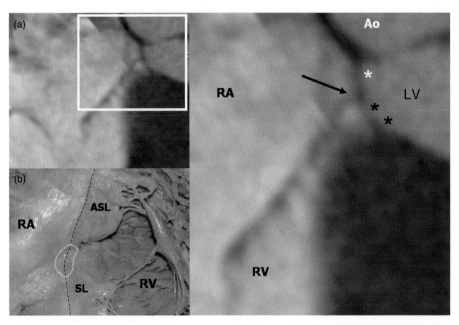

Figure 6.37 (a) Oblique slice with magnified view to show the hinge (arrow in magnified image) of the antero-superior portion of the septal leaflet crossing the membranous septum, dividing it into an atrioventricular portion (white*) and an interventricular portion (**). (b) The septal leaflet displayed to show its hingeline (broken line) crossing the membranous septum (white dotted line). Ao = aorta; RA = right atrium; RV = right ventricle; LV = left ventricle; SL = septal leaflet; ASL = anterior septal leaflet.

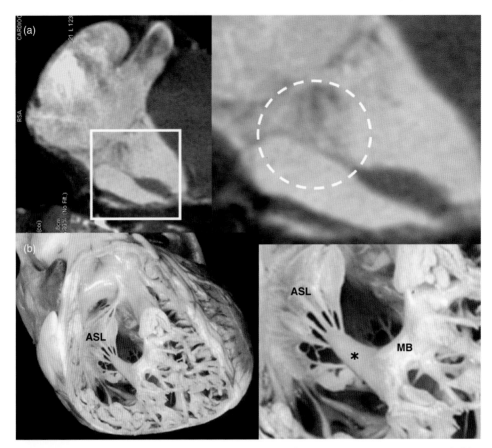

Figure 6.38   Oblique slice and heart specimen viewed from a similar perspective. The anterior papillary muscle (∗) arises from the moderator band (MB) and has fan-like cords. ASL = anterior septal leaflet.

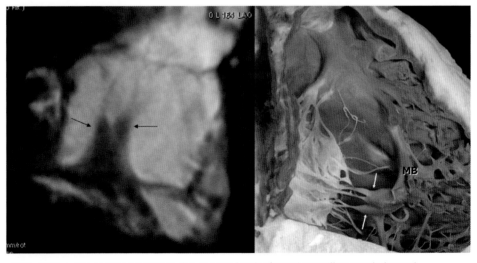

Figure 6.39   Oblique slice and heart specimen showing two heads of anterior papillary muscle (arrows). MB = moderator band.

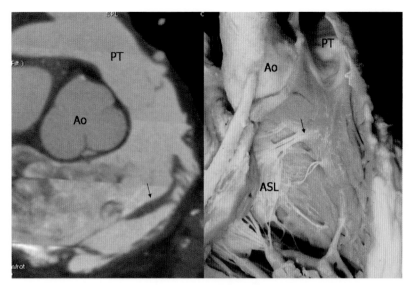

Figure 6.40   Oblique slice and heart specimen showing the medial papillary muscle (arrow). Ao = aorta; ASL = anterior septal leaflet; PT = pulmonary trunk.

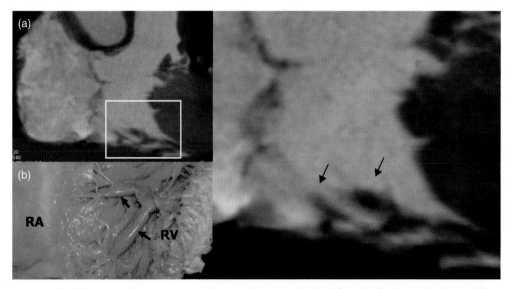

Figure 6.41   (a) Oblique slice showing small papillary muscles supporting the inferior leaflet (arrows in the magnified image). (b) The heart specimen shows two small papillary muscles (arrows). RA = right atrium; RV = right ventricle.

and lifts it above the level of the ventricular septum. Being in an elevated position, the pulmonary valve can be harvested intact for use in surgery to replace the patient's aortic valve (the Ross procedure). The ventricular septum is not transgressed when the pulmonary valve is detached (see also Chapter 4) (Fig. 6.45). The proximal part of the infundibulum blends into the ventriculo-infundibular fold on the medial aspect and forms the supraventricular crest that separates the tricuspid from pulmonary valves (see also Chapter 4) (Figs. 6.46 and 6.47). Because the subpulmonary infundibulum is not a septal structure, it is more accurate to describe its walls as free wall and paraseptal wall when carrying out catheter ablations for right ventricular outflow tract ventricular tachycardia. It is also important to appreciate that the paraseptal

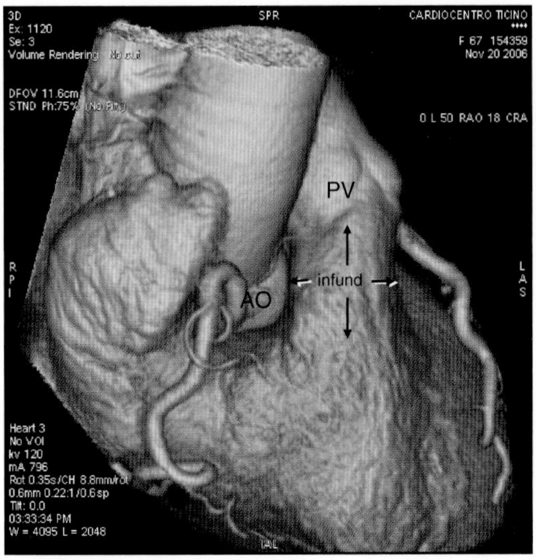

Figure 6.42 3D volume rendering modality. The pulmonary valve (PV) is anterior, superior, and slightly to the left of the aortic valve (AO). A muscular tube, the infundibulum (infund), supports the pulmonary valve.

component lies anterior to the proximal portions of the left and right coronary arteries (Fig. 6.48a).

Each valve consists of three approximately equal-sized semilunar leaflets that are attached by semicircular hingelines to the junctional area comprising muscular infundibulum and arterial wall. Similarly to the aorta, this valve does not have an annulus in the traditional sense of a ring-like attachment. The leaflets have semilunar attachments (hingelines) that cross the circular ventriculo-arterial (muscular and arterial wall) junction (Fig. 6.48b). Like the aortic valve, the hingelines form a crown shape that has three prongs. In this crown configuration, the tips of the prongs between the hingelines of adjacent leaflets are termed the interleaflet fibrous triangles. The sinutubular junction is a circular line that can be drawn, figuratively speaking, to join the tips of the prongs, and it marks the juncture between the sinusal and tubular portions of the pulmonary trunk (Figs. 6.48 and 6.49). All three sinuses of the pulmonary valve enclose small pieces of the distal subpulmonary infundibulum because the semilunar hingelines of the leaflets cross the ventriculo-arterial junction. These may harbor arrhythmogenic foci that require ablations to be carried out within the pulmonary sinuses.

The pulmonary trunk (main pulmonary artery) starts from the pulmonary valve. It passes to the left

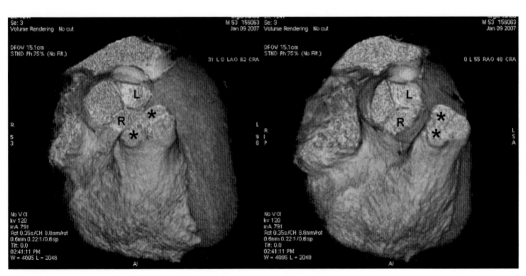

Figure 6.43 3D volume rendering modality. Cranial perspectives. Note the obliquity of the relationship between the aortic and pulmonary valves. Two sinuses of the pulmonary valve (∗∗) "face" the two coronary sinuses of the aortic valve (R and L).

of and posterior to the aorta and divides into the right and left pulmonary arteries (Fig. 6.50). The left pulmonary artery is shorter and higher than the right pulmonary artery and courses in a more posterior direction. The right pulmonary artery passes behind the ascending aorta and underneath the aortic arch to pass rightward behind the superior vena cava and right upper pulmonary

vein (Fig. 6.51). In its proximal course, the right pulmonary artery passes close to the superior wall of the left atrium. The right and left pulmonary arteries divide into ascending and descending branches. The pulmonary artery branches to both lungs usually follow their corresponding bronchial courses.

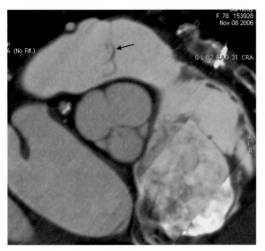

Figure 6.44 Slice showing the heart from atrioventricular plane. Pulmonary leaflets (arrow) are usually thinner than the corresponding aortic leaflets.

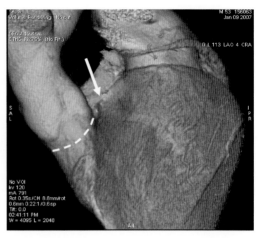

Figure 6.45 3D volume rendering reconstruction after having cropped the aortic root (arrow). The pulmonary valve is supported by the free-standing subpulmonary infundibulum, which is attached only to the right ventricle. The dotted line marks the level at which the pulmonary valve can be detached in its entirety for the Ross procedure.

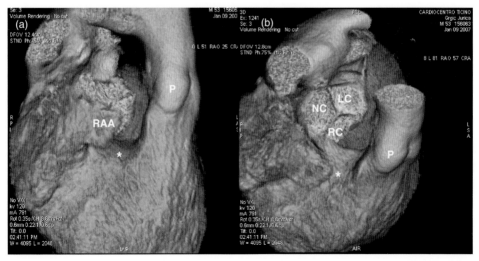

Figure 6.46 3D volume rendering reconstruction after having cropped the aortic root in two slightly different perspectives (a,b). The muscular fold (*) between tricuspid and pulmonary valves is visible. P = pulmonary valve; RAA = right atrial appendage; NC = non-coronary leaflet; LC = left coronary leaflet; RC = right coronary leaflet.

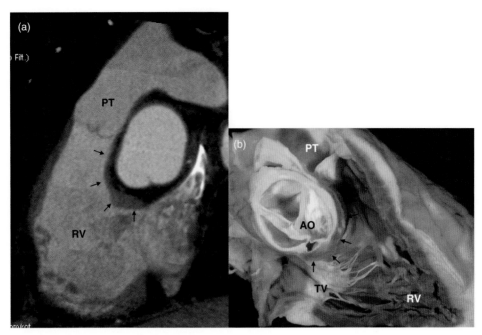

Figure 6.47   (a) Oblique slice showing the muscular fold (arrows) between tricuspid and pulmonary valves. (b) Corresponding cut through a specimen viewed from the right. AO = aorta; PT = pulmonary trunk; RV = right ventricle; TV = tricuspid valve.

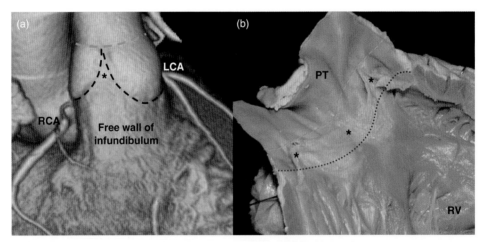

Figure 6.48   (a) 3D volume rendering modality. The crown-shaped attachments of leaflets (black dashed line), the sinutubular junction (blue dashed line) and the anterior fibrous interleaflet triangle (*). Although the paraseptal wall of the muscular infundibulum is hidden behind the free wall in this anterior view, note its proximity to the major coronary arteries. (b) A heart with the pulmonary valve cut longitudinally to display the three leaflets of the pulmonary valve and the interleaflet fibrous triangles (***). The sinutubular junction (blue dashed line) and ventriculo-arterial junction (red dotted line) are circular whereas the attachments (hingelines) of the valvar leaflets form a crown shape. LCA = left coronary artery; RCA = right coronary artery; PT = pulmonary trunk; RV = right ventricle.

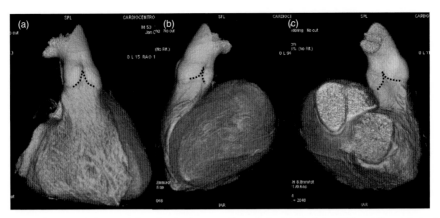

Figure 6.49   3D volume rendering modality after having cropped the aorta and the right and left atria. All three interleaflet triangles (between dotted lines) are shown: the anterior (a), the lateral (b) and the posterior (c). The posterior triangle is adjacent to the aorta.

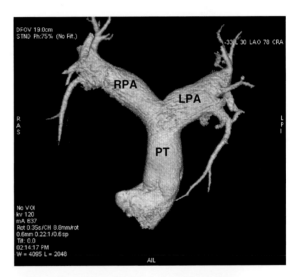

Figure 6.50   3D electronic cast of pulmonary trunk and its branches (see text). PT = pulmonary trunk; RPA = right pulmonary artery; LPA = left pulmonary artery.

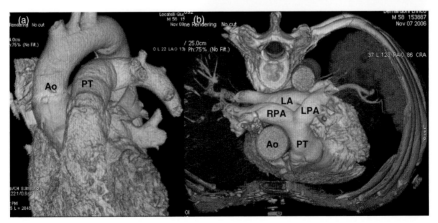

Figure 6.51   Electronic cast from anterior (a) and cranial (b) perspectives showing the relationship between the pulmonary trunk and its branches to the aorta (see text). Ao = aorta; LA = left atrium; LPA = left pulmonary artery; RPA = right pulmonary artery; PT = pulmonary trunk.

Suggested reading

Anderson RH, Ho SY, Brecker SJ. Anatomic basis of cross-sectional echocardiography. *Heart* 2001;85:716–720.

Ho SY. Anatomy of the mitral valve. *Heart* 2002;88:5–10.

Ho SY, McCarthy KP, Josen M, Rigby ML. Anatomic-echocardiographic correlates: an introduction to normal and congenitally malformed hearts. *Heart* 2001; 86(Suppl 2):II3–II11.

Ho SY, Nihoyannopoulos P. Anatomy, echocardiography, and normal right ventricular dimensions. *Heart* 2006;92:i2–i13.

Merrick AF, Yacoub MH, Ho SY, Anderson RH. Anatomy of the muscular subpulmonary infundibulum with regard to the Ross procedure. *Ann Thorac Surg* 2000; 69:556–561.

Perloff JK, Roberts WC. The mitral valve apparatus. Functional anatomy of mitral regurgitation. *Circulation* 1972;46:227–239.

Ranganathan N, Lam JHC, Wigle ED *et al.* Morphology of the human mitral valve. II. The valve leaflets. *Circulation* 1970;41:459–467.

Stamm C, Anderson RH, Ho SY. Clinical anatomy of the normal pulmonary root compared with that in isolated pulmonary valvular stenosis. *J Am Coll Cardiol* 1998;31:1420–1425.

Sutton JP, Ho SY, Anderson RH. The forgotten interleaflet triangles: a review of the surgical anatomy of the aortic valve. *Ann Thorac Surg* 1995;59:419–427.

Underwood MJ, Khoury GE, Deronck D, Glineur D, Dion R. The aortic root: structure, function, and surgical reconstruction. *Heart* 2000;83;376–380.

CHAPTER 7

The Cardiac Septum

Atrial septum

The right atrium (RA) is limited medially by its septal surface, which is formed by the fossa ovalis and its surrounding rim (Figs. 7.1a,b and 7.2a–c). The rim (limbus) often appears as thicker muscle surrounding an oval-shaped depression (the fossa), which has as its floor a thin valve that lies on the left atrial aspect.

The superior rim of the atrial septum, although often referred to as the septum secundum, is actually an extensive infolding of the atrial wall between the venous component of the right atrium and the right pulmonary veins (Fig. 7.3). Externally, this infolding (also called Waterson's groove) is filled with epicardial fat and frequently contains the artery supplying the sinus node. Surgical dissections into this groove allow the surgeon to enter the left atrium for inspection or repair of the mitral valve without transgressing into the right atrium. Lipomatous hypertrophy of atrial septum is characterized by an excessive accumulation of adipose tissue in this groove.

The fossa ovalis is completely overlapped by its valve, a flap of tissue that is continuous with the left atrial wall. During fetal life, the valve opens leftward, allowing blood to flow from the right atrium into the left atrium through its aperture, known as the foramen ovale. After birth, higher pressures in the left atrium push the valve rightward onto its rim, closing the foramen ovale. The foramen ovale is anatomically closed in about two-thirds of adults due to complete adhesion of the valve to its rim. In the remaining one-third

Anatomy of the Heart by Multislice Computed Tomography.
By Francesco Fulvio Faletra, Natesa G. Pandian and Siew Yen Ho. Published 2008 by Wiley-Blackwell Publishing, ISBN: 978-1-4051-8055-9.

of adults incomplete adhesion of the valve to its muscular rim results in a crevice-like patency at its antero-superior margin that is described as a patent foramen ovale. There remains a potential source for right-to-left shunt through a patent foramen. Stretching of the septum when the atria are markedly dilated can transform a patent foramen ovale into an acquired atrial septal defect. Furthermore, redundant valve tissue may form an aneurysm of the fossa ovalis.

The true atrial septum, defined as the tissue that separates the adjacent atrial cavities, and which can be removed without exiting the heart, is confined to the thin valve of the fossa ovalis along with the immediate margins of the surrounding muscular rim (Fig. 7.4). This definition has relevance for trans-septal puncture. It is the valve of the fossa ovalis that is the safe target for trans-septal crossing. When observing the atrial septum from the right atrial aspect, a raised area called the aortic mound can be seen anterior to the fossa ovalis. It can give the false impression of being part of the septum. Instead, it is the antero-medial part of the right atrial wall. Importantly, passing a pin (or catheter) through this area does not enter the left atrium but goes into the transverse pericardial sinus that lies behind the aortic root (Fig. 7.4). The inferior rim contains right atrial tissues overlying the musculature of the ventricular septum forming the atrioventricular "sandwich" (see also Chapter 6).

Whereas the right aspect of the septum often is characterized by the crater-like structure of the fossa ovalis, the atrial septum is relatively featureless when viewed from the left atrium (Fig. 7.5). Nevertheless, it is important to note that the free margin of the fossa ovale valve lies immediately behind the anterior wall of the left atrium that abuts the transverse pericardial sinus and through it is the aortic root (Fig. 7.5b,d). When making use

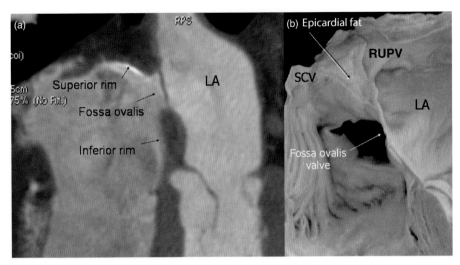

Figure 7.1 (a) Oblique slice and (b) the corresponding anatomic specimen, showing how the true atrial septum is formed by the valve of the foramen and its immediate muscular rim. The infolded superior rim is filled with epicardial fat. LA = left atrium; RUPV = right upper pulmonary vein; SVC = superior vena cave.

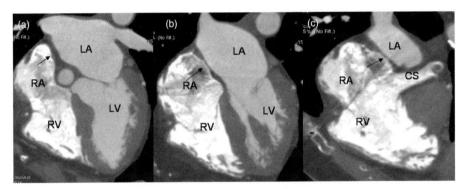

Figure 7.2 Oblique slices showing the atrial septum at different levels: superior rim (a); fossa ovalis (b) and inferior rim (c) (arrow). RA = right atrium; RV = right ventricle; LA = left atrium; LV = left ventricle; CS = coronary sinus.

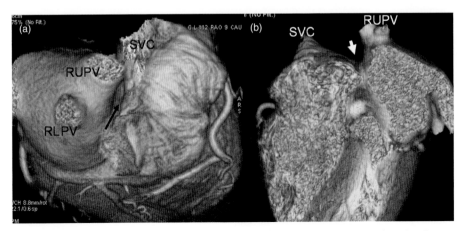

Figure 7.3 3D volume rendering. The arrow indicates the superior infolding between the superior vena cava and the right pulmonary veins; (a) external view from posterior-superior, and (b) "four-chamber cut." RUPV = right upper pulmonary vein; RLPV = right lower pulmonary vein; SVC = superior vena cava.

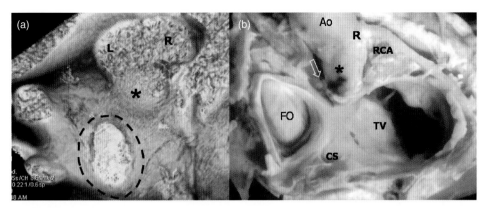

Figure 7.4 (a) 3D volume rendering of atrial septum from the right atrial perspective after having removed the contrast. The dotted line encircles the fossa ovalis. The asterisk points to the non-coronary aortic sinus that abuts against the atrial septum. (b) An anatomic specimen displayed in the same orientation showing the same features. The right atrial walls have been removed, leaving the true atrial septum and without entering the left atrium. The open arrow indicates the transverse pericardial sinus. CS = coronary sinus; FO = fossa ovalis valve; R = right coronary aortic sinus; L = left coronary aortic sinus; RCA = right coronary artery; TV = tricuspid valve; Ao = aorta.

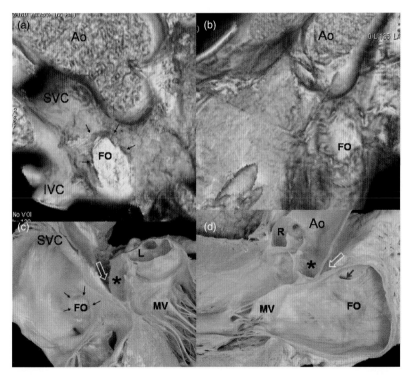

Figure 7.5 3D volume rendering from the same patient as shown in Fig. 7.4 and comparable displays of a heart specimen. The atrial septum is seen from right (a,c) and left (b,d) atrial perspectives. From the right aspect, the septum can be identified by the raised rim of the fossa (arrows) whereas the left aspect is relatively flat. The specimen shows the crevice of the patent foramen ovale (red arrow). The open arrows indicate the transverse pericardial sinus and the asterisks indicate the non-coronary aortic sinus. Ao = aorta; FO = foramen ovale valve; L and R = left and right coronary aortic sinuses, respectively; SVC = superior vena cava; IVC = inferior vena cava; MV = mitral valve.

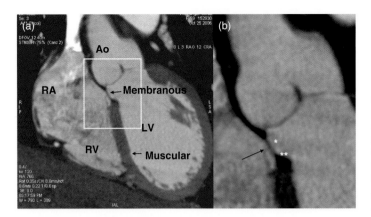

Figure 7.6   (a) The membranous septum and muscular components of the septum. (b) The membranous septum is divided by the septal leaflet of the tricuspid valve (arrow) into atrioventricular (∗) and interventricular (∗∗) components. Ao = aorta; LV = left ventricle; RA = right atrium; RV = right ventricle.

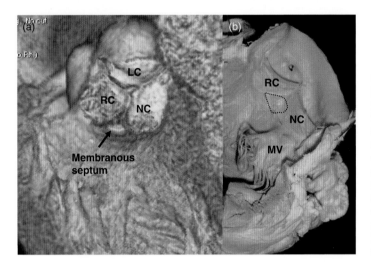

Figure 7.7   3D volume rendering (a) Left ventricle from the left lateral perspective after having removed the contrast. The membranous septum is easily appreciated beneath the right and posterior (non-coronary) aortic leaflets. (b) Heart specimen with the left ventricular outflow tract opened to show the thin area of the membranous septum (within dotted line). LC = left coronary leaflet; NC = non-coronary leaflet; RC = right coronary leaflet; MV = mitral valve.

of a patent foramen ovale to access the left atrium, the proximity of these structures must be borne in mind.

Membranous septum

This is a small component of the cardiac septum but is important on account of its central location in the heart. It is a part of the central fibrous body, the other part being the right fibrous trigone. Because the atrioventricular bundle of the conduction system usually passes between the membranous septum and the crest of the muscular septum, the membranous septum is a useful landmark for its location. The membranous septum is located immediately below the right and posterior (non-coronary) aortic sinuses (Figs. 7.6 and 7.7).

On the right aspect, the hingeline of the septal leaflet of the tricuspid valve divides the membranous septum into an interventricular and an atrioventricular component (Fig. 7.6b) (see also Chapter 5 – tricuspid valve). The atrioventricular component lies between the right atrium and the left ventricle. Perimembranous ventricular septal defects (also known as membranous defects) are deficiencies of the cardiac septum in the environs of the membranous septum.

Ventricular septum

The ventricular (or interventricular) septum separates the left and right ventricles. It is almost entirely composed of muscle other than at the site of the membranous septum.

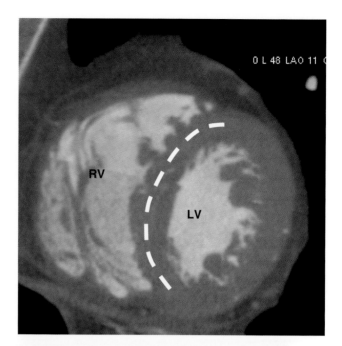

Figure 7.8 Oblique slice. Short-axis section through mid-ventricular cavity to show the normal curvature of the muscular septum. RV = right ventricle; LV = left ventricle.

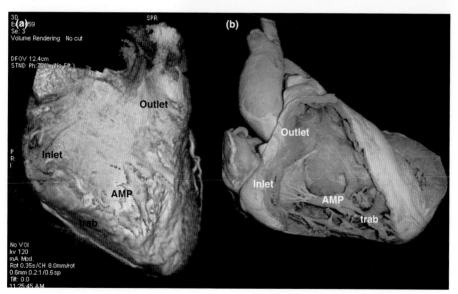

Figure 7.9 3D volume rendering (a) The ventricular septum viewed from the right ventricular perspective after having cropped the antero-lateral wall and removed the contrast. The upper portion of the right ventricular outlet (arrow) is not a septal structure. (b) A corresponding view of a heart specimen. AMP = anterior papillary muscle; trab = trabecular portion.

It is a non-planar structure. Under normal loading conditions it has a convex shape toward the right ventricle (Fig. 7.8). Each ventricle can be described as having three portions: the inlet, trabecular and outlet portions (Figs. 7.9 and 7.10).

Correspondingly, the muscular ventricular septum may be conceptualized as having three portions, but there are important anatomic considerations. Firstly, there is no discrete part that can be designated an outlet septum in the normally structured

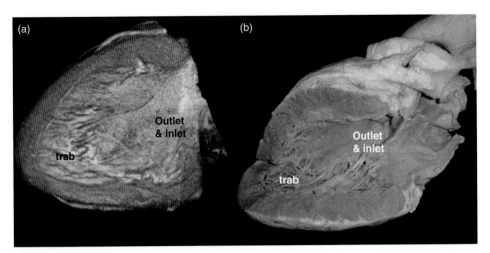

Figure 7.10   (a) 3D volume rendering. The septum viewed from a left lateral perspective after having cropped the lateral wall and removed the contrast. (b) Heart specimen in similar orientation showing the adjoining inlet and outlet portions. trab = trabecular portion.

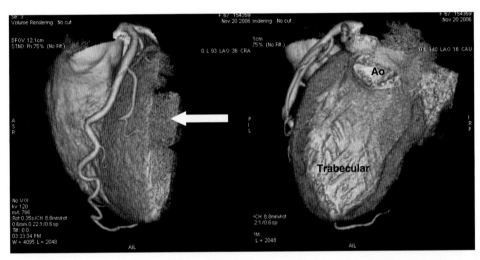

Figure 7.11   3D volume rendering. Proper cropping along with contrast cleaning allows evaluation of the left ventricular surface of the ventricular septum. The trabecular septum is easily appreciated (see also Fig. 7.5b). Ao = aorta.

heart. A large part of the outlet is the subpulmonary muscular infundibulum and the remainder is the supraventricular crest (Fig. 7.9). Secondly, the inlet portion in the right ventricle relates to the tricuspid valve but on the left ventricular aspect the same portion relates to the overlapping left ventricular inlet and outlets (Fig. 7.10).

The *inlet portion* as viewed from the right ventricle is infero-posterior to the membranous septum. It begins at the hingeline (annulus) of the tricuspid valve and ends at the insertions of the papillary muscles (Fig. 7.9). The *outlet portion*, or infundibular part, separates the right from the left ventricular outflow tracts. The *trabecular portion* is the apical part of the ventricular septum. It is characterized by irregularly arranged trabeculations compared with the other portions of the septum (Fig. 7.11).

Suggested reading

Ho SY, Anderson RH, Sanchez-Quintana D. Atrial structure and fibres: morphological basis of atrial conduction. *Cardiovasc Res* 2002;54:325–336.

Lima JA, Guzman PA, Yin FC *et al.* Septal geometry in the unloaded living human heart. *Circulation* 1986;74(3):463–468.

Hagen PT, Scholz DG, Edwards WD. Incidence and size of patent foramen ovale during the first 10 decades of life: an autopsy study of 965 normal hearts. *Mayo Clin Proc* 1984;59:17–20.

Schwinger ME, Gindea AJ, Freedberg RS, Kronzon I. The anatomy of the interatrial septum: a transesophageal echocardiographic study. *Am Heart J* 1990;119:1401–1405.

Shirani J, Roberts WC. Morphology features of fossa ovalis membrane aneurysm in the adult and its clinical significance. *J Am Coll Cardiol* 1995;26:466–471.

CHAPTER 8

Coronary Artery Anatomy

The coronary arterial tree is divided into three segments. Two of these (the left anterior descending artery and the circumflex artery) arise from a common stem whereas the third segment is the right coronary artery. The coronary arteries (as the name suggests) form a crown around the heart. The anterior crown follows the interventricular sulcus (groove) and comprises the left anterior descending and the right posterior descending coronary arteries (Fig. 8.1). The posterior crown follows the atrioventricular sulcus and is formed by the right coronary artery and its postero-lateral branches, and the left main artery and the circumflex artery (Fig. 8.2).

The right and left coronary arteries originate from their respective aortic sinuses. The ostia usually are located in the upper third of the sinuses of Valsalva, although individual hearts may show marked variability (Figs. 8.3 and 8.4). The right coronary artery emerges at nearly right angles to the aortic wall whereas the left coronary artery takes an acute angle (Fig. 8.4). Because of the oblique plane of the aortic valve, the orifice of the left coronary artery is superior and posterior to that of the right coronary artery (Fig. 8.5).

The major epicardial coronary arteries running in the interventricular or atrioventricular grooves are embedded in epicardial fat. This arrangement is thought to be protective against the friction caused by the cardiac contraction (Fig. 8.6).

The *dominance* of the coronary circulation (right versus left) refers to the artery from which the posterior descending artery originates, not

Anatomy of the Heart by Multislice Computed Tomography.
By Francesco Fulvio Faletra, Natesa G. Pandian and
Siew Yen Ho. Published 2008 by Wiley-Blackwell Publishing,
ISBN: 978-1-4051-8055-9.

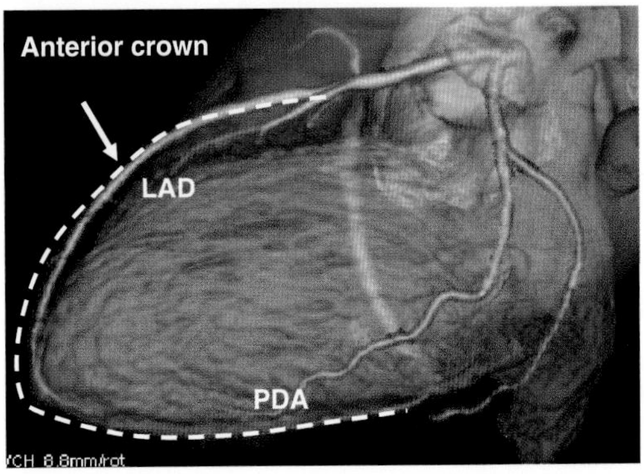

Figure 8.1 Electronic casts with left and right coronary arteries in "transparency" modality. The coronary arteries form posterior and anterior crowns around the heart. The anterior crown (dashed line) comprises the left anterior descending artery (LAD) and the left posterior descending artery (PDA) and follows the interventricular sulcus.

the absolute mass of myocardium perfused by the left or right coronary arteries. Reciprocity exists between the right and left coronary arteries: a large distribution of one takes place at the cost of the other. Variations of this nature have the greatest implication with regard to the blood supply of the crux and the posterior interventricular sulcus.

In approximately 85% of individuals, the right coronary gives rise to the atrioventricular nodal artery, the posterior descending artery and the postero-lateral left ventricular branches, a pattern described as *right dominance*. These branches supply the atrioventricular node, the inferior wall of the left ventricle and the inferior part of the interventricular septum (Fig. 8.7).

In nearly 5–10% of cases there is a *left dominance*: the left postero-lateral branches, the atrioventricular nodal artery and the posterior descending artery originate from the terminal part of the left

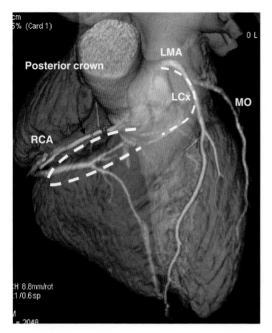

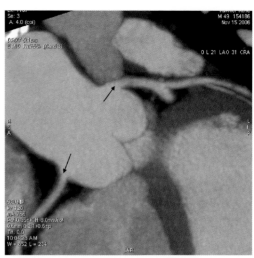

Figure 8.4   The maximal intensity projection (MIP) projection. Oblique view. The image shows how both orifices of coronary arteries originate from the upper part of the aortic sinuses near the sinutubular junction. Note the nearly right-angled take-off of the right coronary artery compared with the acute angle of the left coronary artery.

Figure 8.2   The right and the circumflex coronary arteries lie in the atrioventricular sulcus and form the posterior crown. RCA = right coronary artery; LMA = left main artery; LCx = left circumflex artery; MO = obtuse marginal branch.

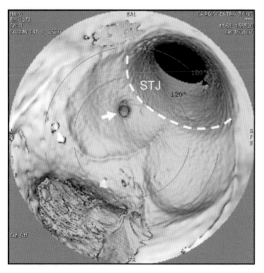

Figure 8.3   3D virtual endoscopy showing endocardial surface of left and posterior aortic sinuses from the ventricular perspective. The orifice of the left coronary artery is located in the upper third of the sinus (arrow). STJ = sinutubular junction.

circumflex artery. Left dominance occurs slightly more frequently in males than females (Fig. 8.8).

In nearly 5% of cases there is a codominance, or *balanced* system, where the right coronary artery gives rise to the posterior descending artery and atrioventricular nodal artery whereas the circumflex artery gives rise to the left postero-lateral branches (Fig. 8.9), or parallel branches from both left and right arteries descend to either side of the interventricular groove and the posterior descending artery is absent.

The left coronary artery

The *left main artery* arises from the left coronary sinus and has an initial diameter of 4–5 mm. It passes behind the pulmonary trunk for 5–10 mm before dividing into the left anterior descending (LAD) artery and left circumflex artery (LCx) (Figs. 8.10a,b and 8.11).

In some hearts, an artery, which is usually called ramus intermedius (intermediate branch), originates from the angle between the division of the anterior descending and the circumflex arteries. This creates the appearance of a trifurcation of the

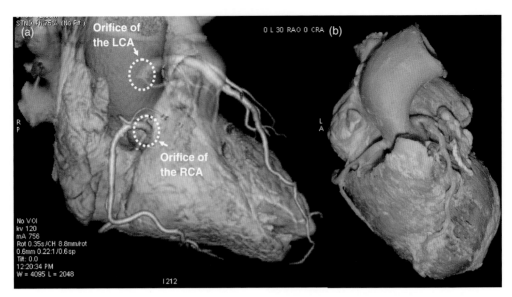

Figure 8.5 (a) Electronic casts with left and right coronary arteries in "transparency" modality showing the orifice of the left coronary artery (LCA) superior and posterior to that of the right coronary artery (RCA). (b) Dissection of a heart specimen showing the same arrangement as the electronic cast.

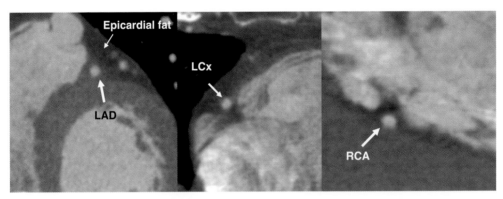

Figure 8.6 Three slices showing how all the major epicardial coronary arteries in the interventricular or atrioventricular grooves pass within epicardial fat.

LAD = left anterior descending artery; LCx = left circumflex artery; RCA = right coronary artery.

main trunk. The ramus intermedius has a course similar to that of the first diagonal branch of the LAD artery or to that of the obtuse marginal branch of the left circumflex artery depending on whether it supplies the anterior or the lateral wall of the left ventricle (Fig. 8.12a,b).

The *left anterior descending* (or *interventricular*) *coronary artery* continues directly from the bifurcation of the left main artery coursing anteriorly and inferiorly in the anterior interventricular groove to the apex of the heart (Fig. 8.13a,d). In many cases it continues around the apex to ascend the apical part of the posterior interventricular groove (Fig. 8.14a,b).

The left anterior descending artery gives rise to the diagonals, the septal perforators and the right ventricular branches. The diagonals, which may be two to six in number, course leftward to supply the antero-lateral wall of the left ventricle. The first diagonal generally is the largest. These branches are numbered as they arise from the artery (Fig. 8.15).

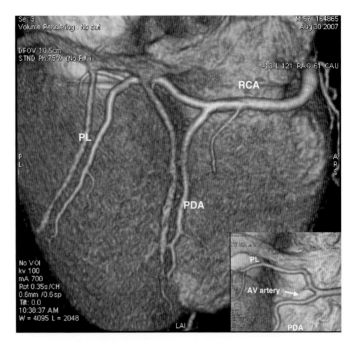

Figure 8.7 3D volume rendering of the inferior surface of the heart showing "right dominance:" both the posterior descending artery (PDA) and left postero-lateral branches (PL) originate from the right coronary artery. Inset shows the atrioventricular (AV) nodal artery originating from a postero-lateral branch (PL) near the bifurcation. RCA = right coronary artery.

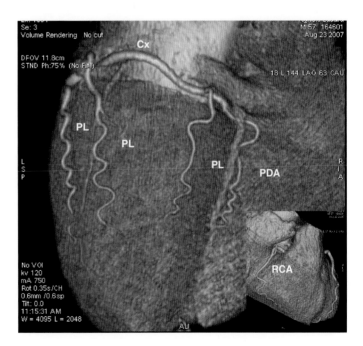

Figure 8.8 3D volume rendering of the inferior surface of the heart showing "left dominance:" the posterior descending artery (PDA) and left postero-lateral branches (PL) originate from the circumflex artery (Cx). Inset shows a short right coronary artery (RCA) terminating at the acute margin.

The septal perforators curve down perpendicularly into the ventricular septum. Typically there are three to five septal perforators; the first one is the largest and commonly originates just beyond the takeoff of the first diagonal. The first septal perforator supplies blood to the atrioventricular (His) bundle and proximal left bundle branch of the conduction system (Fig. 8.16a,b).

Right ventricular branches, which may not always be present, supply blood to the anterior surface of the right ventricle (Fig. 8.17). They course right-ward when they take off from the anterior descending coronary artery.

The *left circumflex coronary artery* (*LCx*) arises from the left main coronary artery nearly at right angles to the LAD. It courses along the left atrio-ventricular groove, and in 85–95% of subjects terminates near the obtuse margin of the left

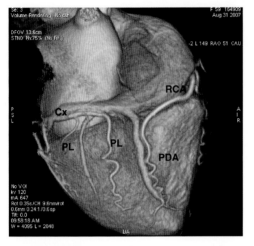

Figure 8.9 3D volume rendering of the inferior surface of the heart showing a "codominance:" the posterior descending artery (PDA) originates from the right coronary artery (RCA) whereas the left postero-lateral branches (PL) originate from the circumflex artery (Cx).

ventricle (Fig. 8.18a,b). In its first segment the vessel courses under the left atrial appendage (Fig. 8.19). In 5–10% of patients it continues around the atrioventricular groove to the crux of the heart to give rise to the posterior descending artery (left dominance: see Fig. 8.8). The primary branches of the left circumflex coronary artery are the left marginal branches or obtuse mar-ginal branches. These vessels supply blood to the lateral aspect of the left ventricular wall, includ-ing the postero-medial papillary muscle. Often the first left marginal branch is larger and longer (therefore clinically more important) than the atrioventricular course of the artery (Fig. 8.20). Additional branches supply blood to the left atrium (Fig. 8.18b) and, in nearly 40% of hearts, the sinus node (Fig. 8.21). When the circumflex coronary artery supplies the posterior descend-ing artery, it usually supplies the atrioventricular node also.

The right coronary artery

The right coronary artery (RCA) arises from the right coronary sinus of the aorta. It courses between the right ventricular outflow tract and the right atrial appendage (RAA) and then runs into the right atrioventricular groove (Fig. 8.22a–d) (see also Video clip 9, Right coronary artery ⓞ).

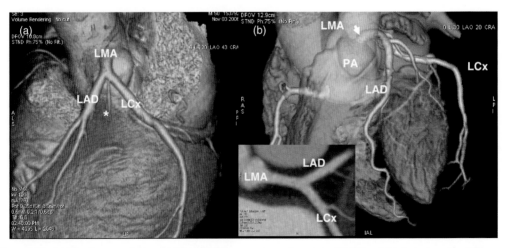

Figure 8.10 (a) 3D volume rendering, (b) 3D transparency modality and (inset) curved multiplan reconstruction of the left main coronary artery (LMA) and its bifurcation into the left anterior descending artery (LAD) and left circumflex artery (LCx). Panel (b) shows how the LMA runs behind the pulmonary artery (PA). The asterisk indicates a small ramus intermedius.

In its very proximal portion, it gives rise to the conus (infundibular) artery, which passes superiorly and medially to supply the infundibulum of the right ventricle (Fig. 8.23).

The *sinus node artery* arises from the right coronary artery in nearly 60% of cases. In most cases the vessel runs in the anterior or superior parts of the interatrial groove to reach the node (Fig. 8.24) by passing in front of or behind the junction between the superior caval vein and the right atrium.

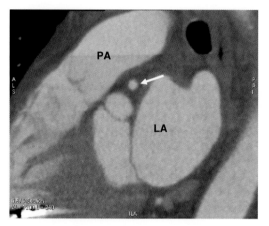

Figure 8.11 Axial projection showing the LMA surrounded by epicardial fat between the body of the left atrium and the pulmonary artery. LA = left atrium; PA = pulmonary artery.

The *right marginal branches* run along the acute margin of the heart. These vessels supply the anterior free wall of the right ventricle (Fig. 8.25). In 10–20% of cases, one of these acute marginal arteries courses across the diaphragmatic surface of the right ventricle to reach the distal ventricular septum (Fig. 8.26). The distal RCA divides into the posterior descending artery (PDA), the posterior left ventricular branches of the RCA (PLB) and the atrioventricular node artery. The PDA runs in the posterior interventricular groove; it arises from a dominant RCA in 85% of individuals. Adjoining the middle cardiac vein (MCV), the posterior descending artery runs anteriorly in the posterior (inferior) interventricular sulcus (Fig. 8.27). In its distal part the right coronary artery gives rise to the posterior lateral branch (PLB). A variable number of posterior lateral branches arising from the distal part of RCA supply the diaphragmatic surface of the left ventricle (Fig. 8.28). The atrioventricular nodal artery arises from the right coronary artery in 80% of the population. In the remaining 20% it originates from the left coronary artery. It branches off from the right coronary artery on the inferior surface of the heart just distal to the origin of PDA. It supplies the atrioventricular node, the atrioventricular bundle of His and the first part of the bundle branches (Fig. 8.28a,b).

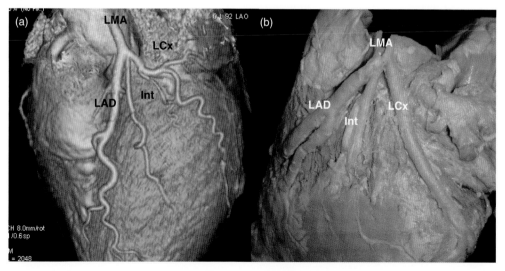

Figure 8.12 (a,b) 3D volume rendering showing the anterior surface of the heart. A large intermediate artery (Int) originates from the angle between the left anterior descending artery (LAD) and the left circumflex artery (LCx). (b) Dissection of a heart specimen showing the same arrangement as the electronic cast. LMA = left main artery.

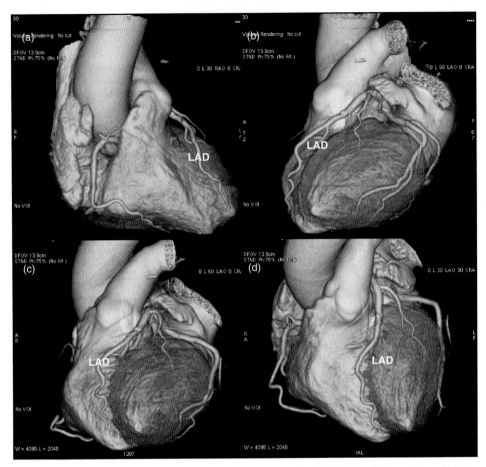

Figure 8.13   3D volume rendering of the left anterior descending artery (LAD) in the four classic angiographic views:
(a) the right oblique 30°; (b) lateral view 90°; (c) left oblique 60° and (d) left cranial view.

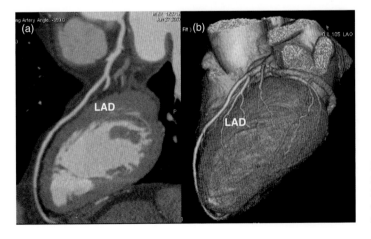

Figure 8.14   (a) Curved multiplanar modality and (b) 3D volume rendering modality showing the entire course of the left anterior descending artery (LAD).

The angiographic view of coronary arteries

Accurate visualization of coronary anatomy by invasive coronary angiography requires coronary injections in multiple views in order to ensure that all coronary segments can be imaged clearly

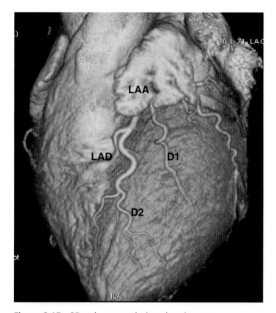

Figure 8.15 3D volume rendering showing two diagonal branches (D1, D2) arising from the left anterior descending artery (LAD). Note how usually the first portion of the LAD is hidden by the left atrial appendage (LAA).

without foreshortening or overlap. Learning the angiographic coronary anatomy might be difficult because of the number of possible projections and the unnatural views of the coronary lumen (without the surrounding imaging of the heart) resulting from various angulations and selective injection of contrast. Compared with the angiographic technique, multislice computed tomography (MSCT) offers the advantage of reconstituting the coronary tree in different standard angiographic views using only one contrast exposure. The best way of representing MSCT angiographic views is the transparency modality. With this modality the coronary tree can be turned to any desired angle (Fig. 8.29) and compared with coronary angiograms. Examples of the most common coronary angiographic views and the corresponding MSCT images are illustrated herein.

The left coronary artery

Antero-posterior projection (Fig. 8.30). The image intensifier is directly over the patient, with the beam perpendicular to the patient lying flat on the x-ray table. The antero-posterior (AP) view displays the left main coronary artery in its entire perpendicular length. In this view, the left anterior descending and left circumflex artery branches are overlapped. Slight right anterior oblique or left anterior oblique angulations may be necessary to clear the density of the vertebrae and the catheter shaft in the thoracic descending aorta.

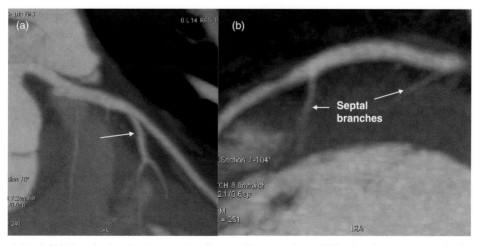

Figure 8.16 (a,b) MIP projection showing septal perforators. These vessels supply blood to the anterior two-thirds of the ventricular septum.

The right anterior oblique projection caudally angulated [*RAO (right anterior oblique) 30°, caudal 30°*] (Fig. 8.31). The image intensifier is to the right side of the patient. The RAO caudal view shows the left main coronary artery bifurcation from a view perpendicular to the left anterior oblique

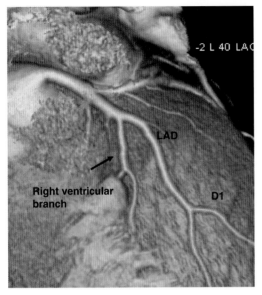

Figure 8.17   3D volume rendering showing a right ventricular branch arising from the left anterior descending artery (LAD).

(LAO)/cranial angle. The origin and course of the circumflex/obtuse marginal, intermediate branch and proximal left anterior descending segment are well seen. This view is one of the best views for visualization of the circumflex artery. The left anterior descending artery beyond the proximal segment is obscured by overlap.

The right anterior oblique (30°) cranial (30°) view (Fig. 8.32). This projection is used to open the diagonal along the mid- and distal left anterior descending arteries. Diagonal branch bifurcations are well visualized. The diagonal branches are projected upward. The proximal left anterior descending and circumflex arteries usually are overlapped. Marginals may overlap, and the circumflex artery is foreshortened.

Left anterior oblique projection (45°) cranial angulated (20°) (Fig. 8.33). In the LAO position, the image intensifier is to the left side of the patient. The LAO (left anterior oblique)/cranial view also shows the left main coronary artery (slightly foreshortened, but perpendicular to the RAO view), left anterior descending, and diagonal branches. Septal and diagonal branches are separated clearly. The circumflex and marginals are foreshortened and overlapped. The LAO angle should be set so that the left anterior descending course is parallel to the

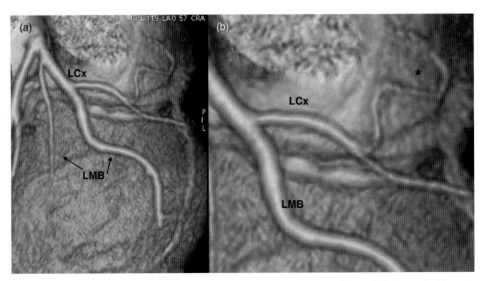

Figure 8.18   3D volume rendering. (a) The left circumflex artery (LCx) and arrows indicate the left marginal branches (LMB). (b) A magnified image showing a left atrial branch (*).

spine and stays in a "lucent wedge" bordered by the spine and the curve of the diaphragm. Cranial angulation tilts the left main coronary artery down and permits view of the left anterior descending/circumflex bifurcation.

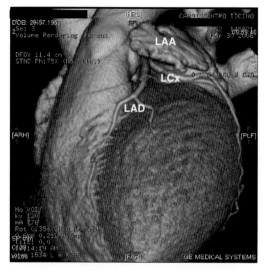

Figure 8.19   3D volume rendering. In its first segment the left circumflex artery (LCx) courses under the left atrial appendage (LAA). LAD = left anterior descending artery.

The LAO lateral view (LAO 90° cranial 0°) (Fig. 8.34). This projection best shows the mid- and distal left anterior descending artery. The left anterior descending and circumflex arteries are well separated. Diagonals usually are overlapped and the intermediate branch course is well visualized. This projection also provides the best look at the anatomosis of a left internal mammary graft to the mid-distal LAD (see Chapter 10).

The right coronary artery

The LAO view (LAO 60°, cranial 0°) shows the origin and the entire length of the right coronary artery, and the posterior descending artery (PDA) bifurcation (crux) (Fig. 8.35).

The lateral view (90° cranial 0°) also shows the right coronary artery origin (especially in those with more anteriorly oriented orifices) and the mid-right coronary artery. The posterior descending artery and postero-lateral branches are foreshortened (Fig. 8.36).

The most frequent anatomic variants

Today, with the widespread use of new imaging techniques for diagnosis and the development of

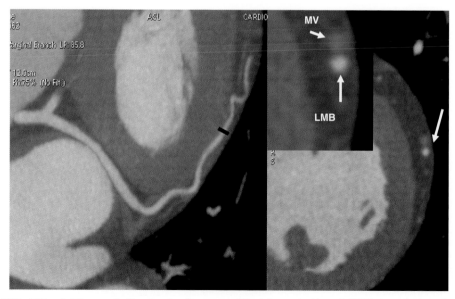

Figure 8.20   MIP and oblique projection showing the course of the left marginal branch (LMB) along the lateral wall of the left ventricle (arrow). In the magnified image the corresponding vein (MV) can also be appreciated.

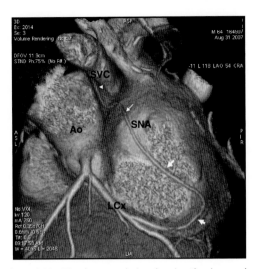

Figure 8.21   3D volume rendering showing the sinus node artery (SNA) arising from the circumflex artery. In about 30% of cases there is a left sinus node vascularization. Ao = aorta; LCx = left circumflex artery; SVC = superior vena cava.

non-aggressive treatments, a thorough knowledge of anatomic variation and anomalies is important. There is considerable patient-to-patient variability in size, position and course of the coronary arteries. An anomaly should be defined as any coronary pattern with a feature (number of ostia, proximal course, termination, etc.) "rarely" encountered in the general population. In nearly 1% of cases these anatomic variants are sufficiently divergent to justify describing them as coronary anomalies.

For several decades, diagnosis of coronary artery anomalies was made with angiography. However, conventional angiographic findings allow correct identification of the abnormalities in just barely half of the cases. The reason for this failure may be that coronary artery anomalies are very difficult to visualize at angiography, and even if they are visualized, their course cannot be delineated accurately.

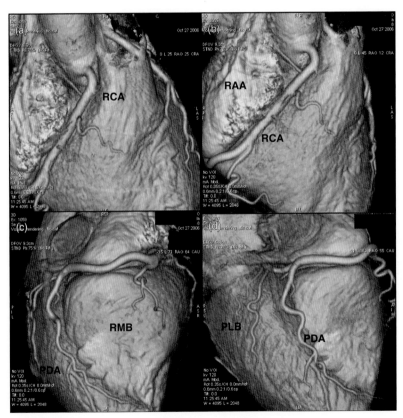

Figure 8.22   3D volume rendering. (a–d) The four panels show the entire course of the right coronary artery and its branches in four different perspectives. RCA = right coronary artery; RAA = right atrial appendage; PDA = posterior descending artery; PLB = postero-lateral branch; RMB = right marginal branch.

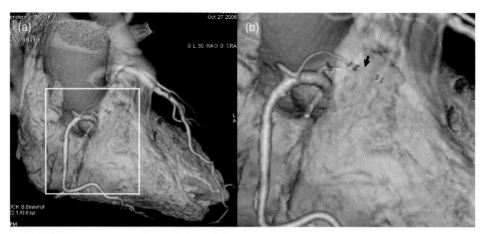

Figure 8.23 (a) 3D transparency modality showing right and left coronary arteries. (b) Magnified image showing the conus artery (arrow).

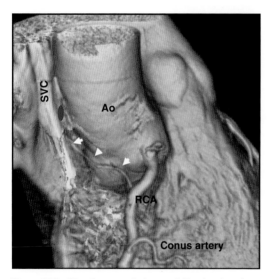

Figure 8.24 3D volume rendering modality showing the course of sinus node artery (arrows) toward the sinus node (red oval). Ao = aorta; RCA = right coronary artery; SVC = superior vena cava.

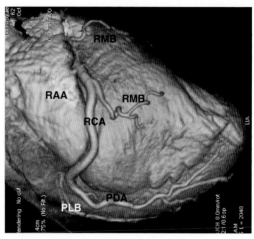

Figure 8.25 3D volume rendering. Right lateral perspective showing the acute margin of the heart. Two right marginal branches (RMB) are visible. RAA = right atrial appendage; RCA = right coronary artery; PDA = posterior descending artery; PLB = postero-lateral branch.

MSCT seems to be superior to coronary angiography in defining the origin and course of anomalous coronary branches. In this part of the chapter we will show some the most frequent coronary anomalies. For a more comprehensive description see the references listed under "Suggested reading."

High take-off. "High take-off" refers to the origin of either the RCA or the LCA at a level well above the junctional zone between its sinus and the tubular part of the ascending aorta. Although high take-off with proximal intramural course of the artery in the aortic wall has been implicated in sudden cardiac death, high take-off usually presents no major clinical problems, but it may cause difficulty in cannulating the vessels during coronary arteriography.

Multiple orifices in the right aortic sinus: the most frequent variation is the presence of an accessory orifice for the conal artery. The orifice of the conal artery is usually in front of the coronary orifice or at the same level. The diameter varies between 0.5 and 1.5 mm (Fig. 8.37).

Multiple orifices in the left aortic sinus: the most frequent variation is the absence of a common trunk of the left coronary artery, which means that the anterior interventricular artery and the circumflex artery have different origins. The prevalence ranges between 0.5% and 1%. This variation may take the form of either two separate, well-defined orifices or a mixed orifice ("shotgun" orifice) (Fig. 8.38). Both left anterior descending artery and circumflex artery are otherwise normal in their distribution pattern. This anomaly does not cause any hemodynamic impairment.

Single coronary artery is the anomalous situation of only one coronary artery arising with a single

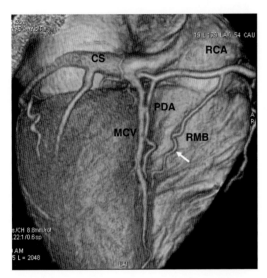

Figure 8.26   3D volume rendering of the inferior view of the heart. Right coronary artery (RCA), posterior descending artery (PDA), right marginal branch (RMB), middle cardiac vein (MCV) and coronary sinus (CS) are visualized. Arrow shows a right marginal branch reaching the diaphragmatic surface of the right ventricle

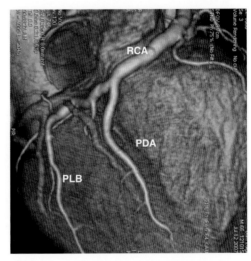

Figure 8.27   3D volume rendering of the inferior view of the heart showing the right coronary artery (RCA), the posterior descending artery (PDA) and the posterior lateral branch (PLB).

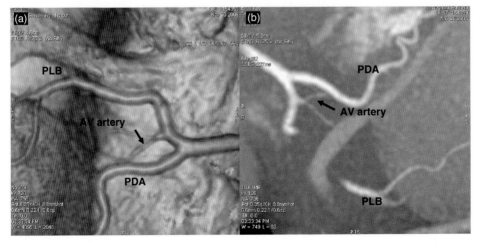

Figure 8.28   (a) 3D volume rendering and (b) MIP slice of the crux showing a small atrioventricular branch (arrow). PDA = posterior descending artery; PLB = posterior lateral branch.

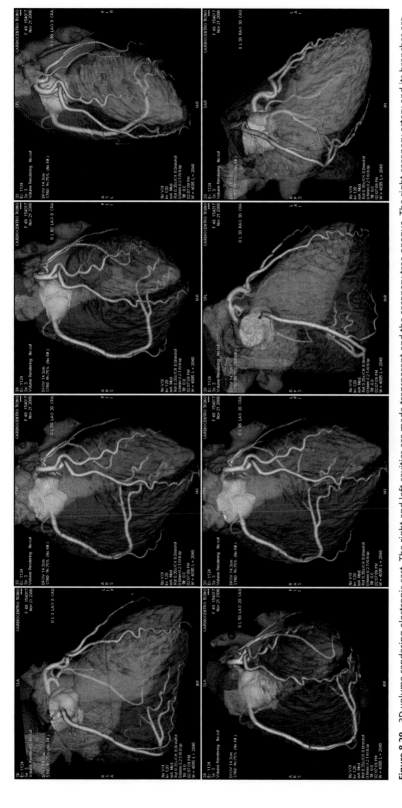

Figure 8.29   3D volume rendering electronic cast. The right and left cavities are made transparent and the coronary tree opaque. The right coronary artery and its branches are shown in any angulation. This composition mimics the most commonly used coronary angiographic projections (see Video clip 10, Coronary Tree 🔵).

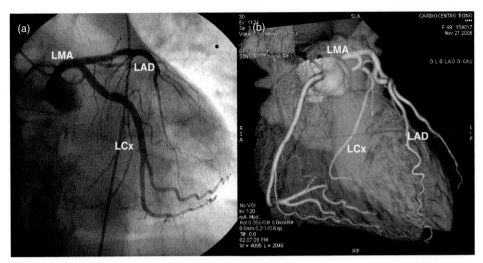

Figure 8.30 (a,b) Frame of the left coronary angiography in antero-posterior projection (a) and the corresponding 3D volume rendering electronic cast. LMA = left main artery; LCx = left circumflex artery; LAD = left anterior descending artery (see text).

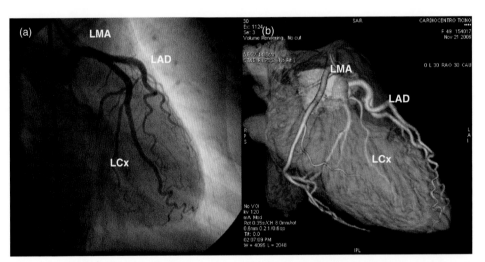

Figure 8.31 (a) Left coronary angiogram in the right anterior oblique (RAO) projection with caudal angulation (RAO 30°, caudal 30°) and (b) the corresponding 3D volume rendering electronic cast. LMA = left main artery; LCx = left circumflex artery ; LAD = left anterior descending artery (see text).

ostium from the aortic trunk (Fig. 8.39). A single coronary artery may either follow the pattern of a normal RCA or LCA, divide into two branches with distributions of the RCA and LCA, or have a distribution different from that of the normal coronary arterial tree. This anomaly is usually compatible with a normal life expectancy.

Anomalous origin. The most common forms of anomalous origin are: the right coronary artery arising from the left coronary sinus; the LCx (or LAD artery) arising from the right coronary sinus; and the LCA or RCA (or a branch of either artery) arising from the non-coronary sinus.

Right coronary artery arising from the left coronary sinus. In this anomaly, the right coronary artery usually passes between aorta and pulmonary artery to reach the right atrioventricular groove. The oblique angle at the juncture with the left

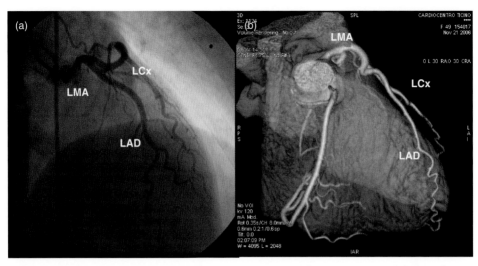

Figure 8.32 (a) Left coronary angiogram in the right anterior oblique (RAO) projection with cranial angulation and (b) the corresponding 3D volume rendering electronic cast. LMA = left main artery; LCx = left circumflex artery; LAD = left anterior descending artery (see text).

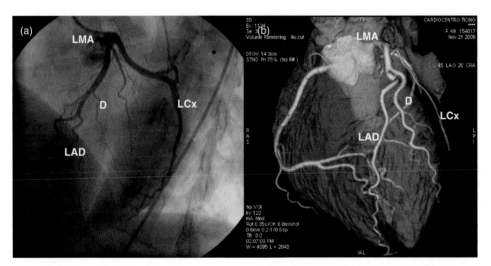

Figure 8.33 (a) Left coronary angiogram in the left anterior oblique projection (LAO) and (b) the corresponding 3D volume rendering electronic cast. LMA = left main artery; LCx = left circumflex artery; LAD = left anterior descending artery; D = diagonal (see text).

coronary sinus produces a slit-like orifice in the aortic wall that might predispose to ischemia and sudden death (Fig. 8.40).

Left circumflex artery arising from the right coronary sinus. The vessel arises from the right sinus of Valsalva as a separate vessel (Fig. 8.41) or as a branch of a single coronary artery in 0.09–0.11% of cases.

Myocardial bridging. Coronary arteries in the human characteristically have an epicardial course. Not infrequently, however, segments of these

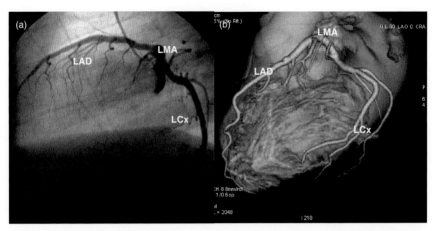

Figure 8.34   (a) Left coronary angiogram in LAO lateral view and (b) the corresponding 3D volume rendering electronic cast. LMA = left main artery; LCx = left circumflex artery ; LAD = left anterior descending artery (see text).

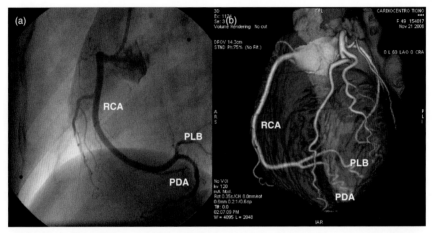

Figure 8.35   (a) Right coronary angiogram in LAO 60° view and (b) the corresponding 3D volume rendering electronic cast. RCA = right coronary artery; PDA = posterior descending artery; PLB = postero-lateral branch (see text).

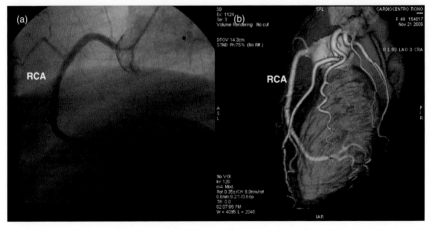

Figure 8.36   (a) Right coronary angiogram in LAO 90° view and (b) the corresponding MSCT view. RCA = right coronary artery (see text)

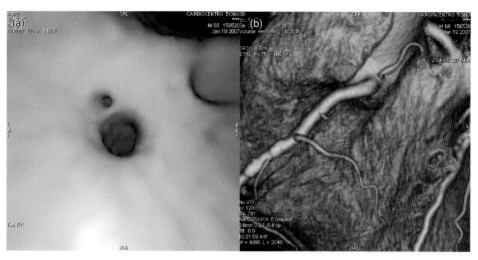

Figure 8.37   (a) 3D virtual endoscopy and (b) 3D volume rendering showing the conus branch originating directly from the aorta.

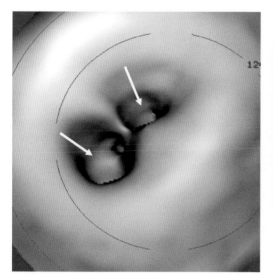

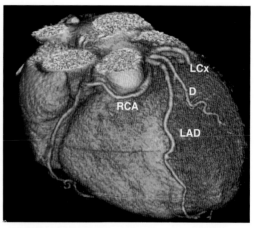

Figure 8.39   3D volume rendering. This anterior view shows only one coronary artery arising from a single ostium in the left coronary sinus. LAD = left anterior descending artery; RCA = right coronary artery; LCx = left circumflex artery; D = diagonal.

Figure 8.38   Virtual endoscopy showing the absence of left main coronary artery. The left anterior descending and the circumflex artery have nearly separate orifices (arrows).

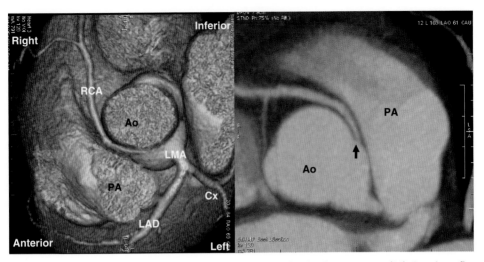

Figure 8.40   3D volume rendering superior view showing the anomalous origin of right coronary artery (RCA) from the left coronary sinus and its course between the aorta (Ao) and pulmonary artery (PA). Cx = circumflex artery; LAD = left anterior descending artery; LMA = left main artery.

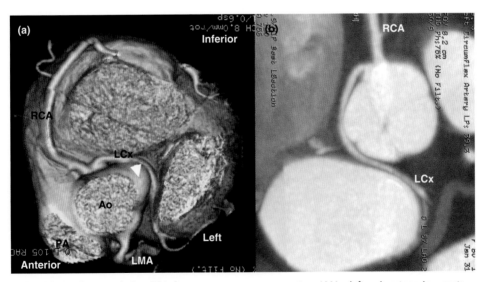

Figure 8.41   (a) 3D volume rendering. (b) Left circumflex artery (LCx) arises from the right coronary sinus taking a retroaortic course. RCA = right coronary artery; LMA = left main artery; Ao = aorta. PA = pulmonary artery.

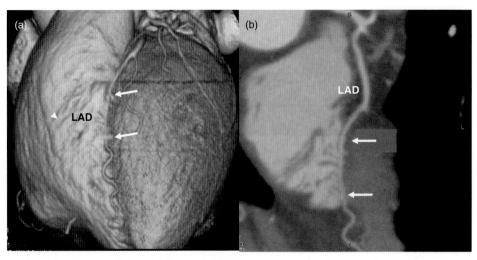

Figure 8.42   (a) 3D volume rendering and (b) curved multiplanar reconstruction showing an intramuscular course (arrows) of the mid-segment of the left anterior descending artery (LAD).

arteries run intramuscularly. This variant is known as myocardial bridging and is most commonly seen in the left anterior descending coronary artery. In most cases, myocardial bridging represents an incidental finding that may be considered a normal variant or a benign coronary anomaly (Fig. 8.42).

Suggested reading

Koizumi M, Kawai K, Honma S, Kodama K. Anatomical study of a left single coronary artery with special reference to the various distribution patterns of bilateral coronary arteries. *Ann Anat* 2000;182(6):549–557.

David NR, Rabin S, Mintzer RA. A pictorial review of coronary artery anatomy on spiral CT. *Chest* 2000;118: 488–491.

Möhlenkamp S, Hort W, Ge J, Erbel R. Update on myocardial bridging. *Circulation* 2002;106:2616–2622.

Nieman K, Oudkerk M, Rensing BJ, *et al.* Coronary angiography with multi-slice computed tomography. *Lancet* 2001;357:599–603.

Von Ludinghausen M. The clinical anatomy of coronary arteries. *Adv Anat Embryol Cell Biol* 2003;167:III–VIII, 1–111.

CHAPTER 9

Coronary Vein Anatomy

The coronary veins including the coronary sinus are used increasingly for different electrophysiological purposes such as cardiac resynchronization therapy, radiofrequency catheter ablation, mapping and defibrillation. Moreover, the anatomic proximity of the coronary sinus to the mitral annulus has been exploited for the development of catheter-based mitral annuloplasty that implants devices inside the coronary sinus to reshape the mitral orifice. The coronary venous circulation comprises the greater cardiac venous system and the smaller cardiac venous system. The latter, also known as Thebesian veins, are thin-walled vessels that open directly into the cardiac chambers. This chapter will focus on the greater venous system, which consists of direct tributaries of the coronary sinus as well as the right coronary vein. We will review the coronary sinus and its main tributaries. Unfortunately, the nomenclature for the tributaries is not standardized to attitudinal orientation.

Greater cardiac venous system

The coronary sinus (CS) is the main channel of venous blood from the myocardium, receiving 85% of coronary venous blood. Following the direction of venous flow, the great cardiac vein ascends the interventricular groove alongside the anterior descending coronary artery. This portion, also described as the anterior interventricular vein, receives numerous branches from the ventricular septum and the anterior aspects of both ventricles. The great cardiac vein then turns leftward to enter the left atrioventricular groove, usually passing underneath the left atrial appendage. Along

Anatomy of the Heart by Multislice Computed Tomography.
By Francesco Fulvio Faletra, Natesa G. Pandian and Siew Yen Ho. Published 2008 by Wiley-Blackwell Publishing, ISBN: 978-1-4051-8055-9.

its course in the atrioventricular groove it usually receives the oblique left obtuse marginal vein (or postero-lateral vein) and the inferior left ventricular vein from the left ventricle, and the oblique vein of Marshall from the left atrium. The latter is normally obliterated to become a ligament. When persistent, it courses as the persistent left superior caval vein. The junction between CS and great cardiac vein is usually taken to be at the level of the insertion of the ligament. The middle cardiac vein passes along the inferior interventricular groove to enter the right atrium close to the CS os. The right (or small) cardiac vein receives tributaries from the right atrium and inferior wall of the right ventricle, courses in the right atrioventricular groove, and enters the right margin of the CS os. It may be larger when it is joined by the acute marginal vein (of Galen) and a number of veins draining the anterior wall of the right ventricle.

Coronary sinus

In the normal heart the CS is a wide venous channel, about 2–3 cm in length; it is often situated slightly proximal to the atrioventricular groove and usually runs along the inferior wall of the left atrium rather than in the atrioventricular groove (Fig. 9.1). It is surrounded to a greater or lesser extent by a muscular coat that often has continuity with the left atrial myocardium. Anatomic observations have shown several degrees of elevation and variable "arched" courses of the coronary sinus (Fig. 9.2). A "normal" position of the coronary sinus in the left posterior atrioventricular groove can be found in only 16% of cases, a slight elevation (1–3 mm) in 12%, a moderate elevation (4–7 mm) in 50% and an extreme elevation (8–15 mm) in 22%. Viewed from above, the coronary sinus describes a gentle curve in the left inferior coronary sulcus, or, when it is elevated as previously described, on the inferior left atrial wall (Fig. 9.3).

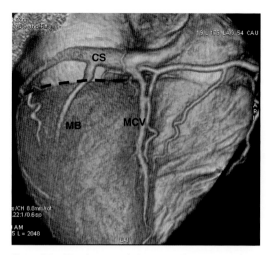

Figure 9.1 3D volume rendering. Note the coronary sinus (CS) is lying on the inferior left atrial wall rather than in the atrioventricular groove (dashed line). MB = marginal branch; MCV = middle cardiac vein.

The position of the CS relative to the atrioventricular groove and to the mitral annulus, and the proximity of the CS to the circumflex artery, should be evaluated prior to procedures in the triage of patients deemed potentially suitable for catheter-based mitral annuloplasty (Figs. 9.2 and 9.3). There is marked variability in the point(s) where the coronary sinus intersects the left circumflex artery and its marginal branches. Appreciation of individual patients' spatial anatomy at overlapping segments between the left circumflex artery and coronary sinus system is therefore a critical factor for the safety of these devices (Fig. 9.4a–d). The CS ostium opens in the right atrium between the opening of the inferior vena cava and the tricuspid orifice at the inferior border of the triangle of Koch (Fig. 9.5). In nearly 80% of cases its orifice is guarded by a semilunar valve, the valve of the coronary sinus (valve of Thebesius) (Fig. 9.6).

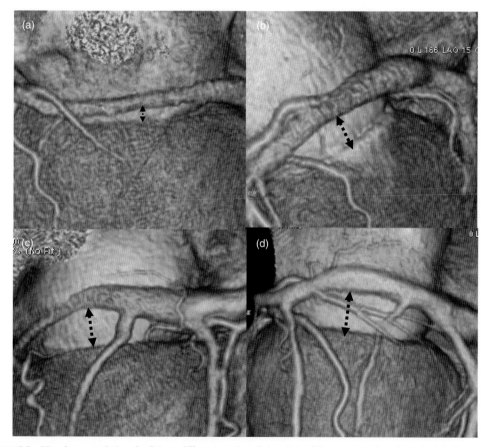

Figure 9.2 3D volume rendering. (a–d) Four different grades of elevation of the coronary sinus from the inferior coronary sulcus to the inferior wall of the left atrium. See Video clip 11, Coronary sinus.

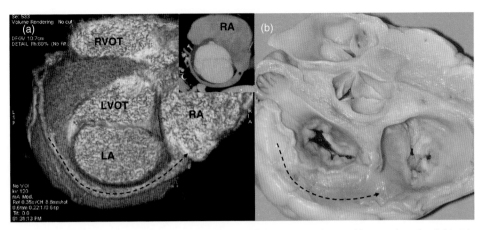

Figure 9.3 (a) 3D volume rendering of coronary sinus (CS). View from above. The great cardiac vein and coronary sinus can be followed (dashed line). Inset: an oblique slice showing the ostium of CS (asterisk). (b) Anatomic specimen with same view from above showing the course of the coronary sinus and its entry into the right atrium (dashed line). LA = left atrium; RA = right atrium; LVOT = left ventricular outflow tract; RVOT = right ventricular outflow tract.

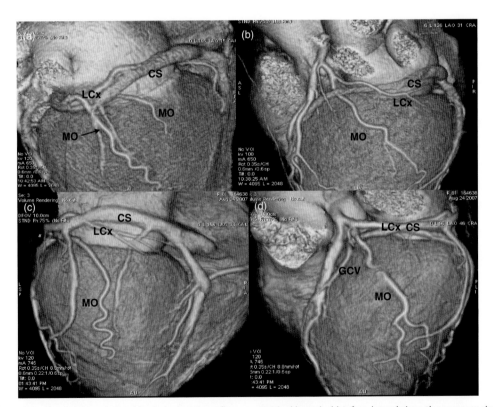

Figure 9.4 The variable relationships between circumflex artery (LCx) and coronary sinus (CS). (a) Infero-lateral view: the coronary sinus crosses over the circumflex artery marginal obtuse branches. (b) Anterior view: the coronary sinus crosses under the circumflex artery and the obtuse marginal branch. (c) Infero-lateral view: the coronary sinus crosses over the circumflex artery and its obtuse marginal branch (MO). (d) Anterior view: the coronary sinus crosses over the circumflex artery and under the obtuse marginal branch. GCV = great cardiac vein.

There are numerous variations in size, length and shape of CS (Fig. 9.7a–c). Rarely, distinctly aneurysmal or diverticular enlargements can occur (Fig. 9.7b).

Great cardiac vein (GCV)(vena cordis magna; left coronary vein)

The GCV begins at the apex of the heart and ascends the anterior interventricular groove alongside the left anterior descending coronary artery to reach the base of the ventricles and then curves leftward toward the left atrioventricular groove. It receives tributaries analogous to the diagonal and septal perforating arteries of the anterior descending coronary artery (Figs. 9.8 and 9.9). Along its course in the basal part of the ventricle it receives tributaries from the left ventricle and left atrium. The GCV may cross over or under the left circumflex artery (Fig. 9.10; see also Fig. 9.4d).

Left marginal veins (postero-lateral cardiac veins)

The left marginal veins drain the lateral and posterior/inferior wall of the left ventricle. The number and size of veins draining the lateral and inferior left ventricular wall are extremely variable. One, two, three or more distinct veins of variable dimensions and course might drain the lateral and inferior wall of the left ventricle (Figs. 9.11–9.13). These veins have been considered recently as conduits for placement of leads for biventricular pacing in the context of cardiac resynchronization therapy.

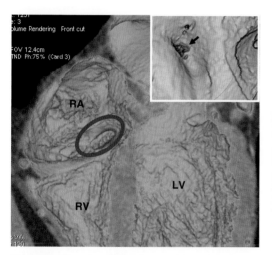

Figure 9.5 3D endocardial surface modality. The red circle marks the ostium of coronary sinus. Inset: image obtained using navigator modality shows the ostium (arrow).

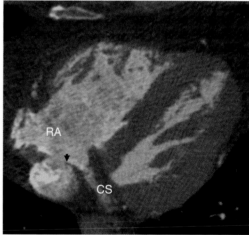

Figure 9.6 Multiplanar oblique view showing the valve of Thebesius (arrow). RA = right atrium; CS = coronary sinus.

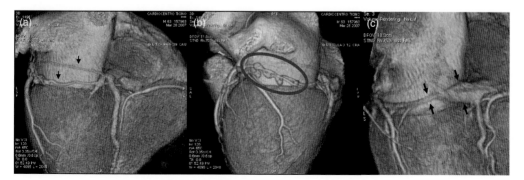

Figure 9.7 3D volume rendering. (a) Inferior view showing a very short CS dividing into two small coronary veins (arrows). (b) Lateral view showing a diverticular arrangement. (c) Inferior view showing an abrupt reduction in size (arrows).

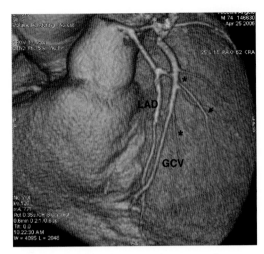

Figure 9.8   3D volume rendering. The great cardiac vein (GCV) in its anterior course runs parallel to the left anterior descending coronary artery (LAD). Asterisks mark tributaries from the anterior left ventricular wall. Arrow marks the first diagonal.

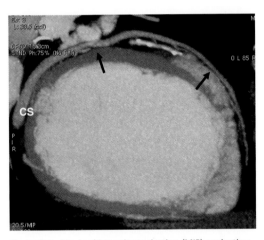

Figure 9.9   Maximal intensity projection (MIP) projection showing the entire course of the great cardiac vein (arrows). CS = coronary sinus.

The phrenic nerve may, on occasion, cross one or more left marginal veins. When it does, direct phrenic nerve stimulation may occur when a pacing lead is inserted in one of these veins (Fig. 9.14).

Middle cardiac vein (MCV) (vena cordis media)

The MCV is the largest proximal tributary to the coronary sinus. The vein commences at the apex of the heart, ascends in the inferior interventricular groove (parallel to the posterior descending

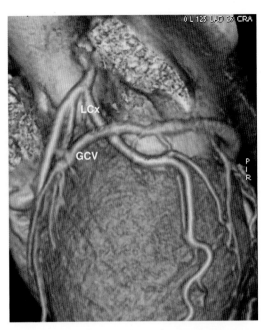

Figure 9.10   3D volume rendering showing the great cardiac vein (GCV) crossing over the left circumflex artery (LCx).

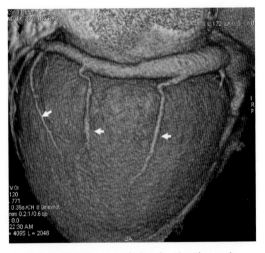

Figure 9.11   3D volume rendering showing three veins along the obtuse margin (arrows).

coronary artery), and terminates in the coronary sinus near to its right extremity (Fig. 9.15). In about 75% of cases, the vein arises as a single vessel and in the remaining 25% as two vessels, sometimes almost equally formed from the superficial network at the cardiac apex (Fig. 9.16). The vein and its tributaries drain the diaphragmatic wall of both left and right

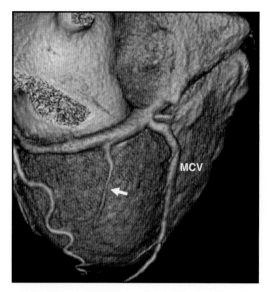

Figure 9.12   3D volume rendering. Only one small posterior left ventricular vein is seen (arrow). Note the larger middle cardiac vein (MCV).

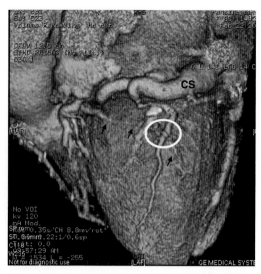

Figure 9.14   3D volume rendering. The course of the left phrenic nerve in the fibrous pericardium is indicated by arrows. The white oval marks the point of crossover. CS = coronary sinus.

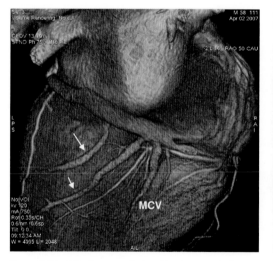

Figure 9.13   3D volume rendering. Two large posterior left ventricular veins (arrows) drain the inferior wall of the left ventricle. MCV = middle cardiac vein.

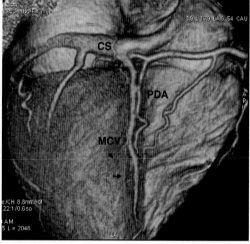

Figure 9.15   3D volume rendering. The middle cardiac vein (MCV) courses parallel to the posterior descending coronary artery (PDA), and ends in the coronary sinus. Arrows mark small distal tributaries. CS = coronary sinus.

ventricles as well the apical area. By means of its septal channels the MCV drains the posterior (inferior) third of the interventricular septum. Rarely anatomic variants of MCV may be encountered. Figure 9.17a shows the MCV lying on the right of the posterior interventricular groove, and Fig. 9.17b shows the MCV entering directly into the right atrium.

Small cardiac vein

The small cardiac vein runs parallel to the distal right coronary artery in the atrioventricular groove draining into either the middle cardiac vein or the coronary sinus just proximal to its ostium (Fig. 9.18). It may also open directly into the right atrium.

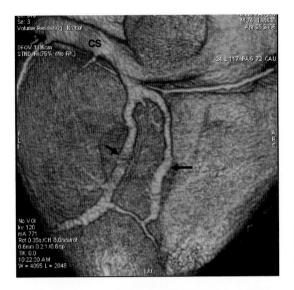

Figure 9.16 3D volume rendering. Two middle cardiac veins (arrows) of the same size ascend from the apex, merging in a single channel before entering into the coronary sinus (CS).

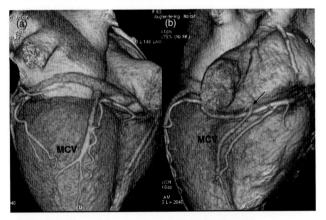

Figure 9.17 (a,b) 3D volume rendering of anatomic variants of middle cardiac vein (MCV).

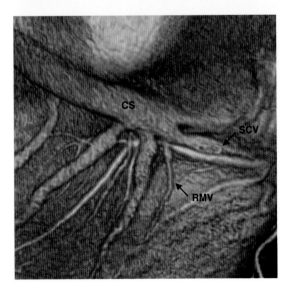

Figure 9.18 3D volume rendering showing a right marginal vein (RMV) joining with the small cardiac vein (SCV) before opening into the coronary sinus (CS) close to the ostium.

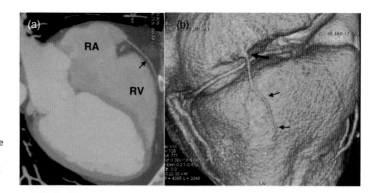

Figure 9.19 (a) MIP slice and (b) 3D volume rendering showing the acute marginal vein entering directly into the right atrium (arrows). RA = right atrium; RV = right ventricle.

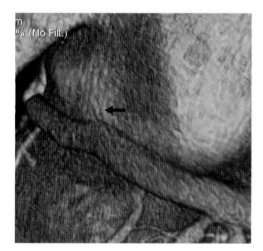

Figure 9.20 3D volume rendering showing Marshall's vein (arrow).

Acute marginal vein

The acute marginal vein ascends along the acute cardiac margin, crosses the atrioventricular groove and opens into the right atrium directly (Fig. 9.19). In some hearts it courses in the right atrioventricular groove toward the cardiac crux, joining with the small cardiac vein to enter close to the ostium of the coronary sinus.

Oblique vein of the left atrium (vein of Marshall)

The oblique vein is a small vessel that descends obliquely on the lateral wall of the left atrium and ends in the coronary sinus near its juncture with the great cardiac vein. It is continuous superiorly with the ligament of the left superior vena cava (ligamentum venae cavae sinistrae; vestigial fold of Marshall) (Fig. 9.20). This small vein has gained interest recently because studies have demonstrated that focal atrial fibrillation can be initiated by an ectopic beat originating from the musculature of this vein, which is heavily innervated.

Suggested reading

Chauvin M, Shah DC, Haissaguerre M *et al.* The anatomic basis of connections between the coronary sinus musculature and the left atrium in humans. *Circulation* 2000;101:647–652.

Doshi RN, Wu T-J, Yashima M *et al.* Relation between ligament of Marshall and adrenergic atrial tachyarrhythmia. *Circulation* 1999;100:876–883.

Gilard M, Mansourati J, Etienne Y *et al.* Angiographic anatomy of the coronary sinus and its tributaries. *Pacing Clin Electrophysiol* 1998;21:2280–2284.

Ho SY, Sanchez-Quintana D, Becker AE. A review of the coronary venous systems: a road less travelled. *Heart Rhythm* 2004;1:107–112.

Ortale JR, Gabriel EA, Iost C *et al.* The anatomy of the coronary sinus and its tributaries. *Surg Radiol Anat* 2001;23:15–21.

Silver MA, Rowley NE. The functional anatomy of the human coronary sinus. *Am Heart J* 1998;115:1080.

von Ludinghausen M. The venous drainage of the human myocardium. *Adv Anat Embryol Cell Biol* 2003;168: I–VIII,1–104.

CHAPTER 10

Coronary Artery Bypass Grafts

Anatomy of internal mammary artery

The internal mammary arteries, also known as the internal thoracic arteries, are paired blood vessels located inside the chest cavity. They arise bilaterally from the lower surface of the first part of the subclavian arteries in 75% of cases, superior and dorsal to the sternal end of the clavicles. In 70% of cases the left internal mammary artery arises on its own, whereas in 30% it arises from a common trunk with other arteries (thyrocervical trunk, suprascapular artery, inferior thyroid artery). The internal mammary arteries run along the inside edge of the sternum (Figs. 10.1 and 10.2), sending off small branches to the bones, cartilage and soft tissues of the chest wall. For reasons that are still unclear, the internal mammary artery is remarkably resistant to cholesterol buildup. It is an elastic artery with a well-formed internal elastic membrane and a thin intima. The left internal mammary artery is also conveniently located near the most important coronary branch, the left anterior descending (Fig. 10.3). The surgeon can transfer the lower end of the left internal mammary artery down to the heart surface to use as a bypass graft to the coronary vessels. Figure 10.4 shows the left internal mammary artery as it appears in the operating room.

Coronary artery bypass grafts

Coronary artery bypass grafts are extra-anatomic bypasses connecting a major arterial branch (normally the ascending aorta and/or the proximal

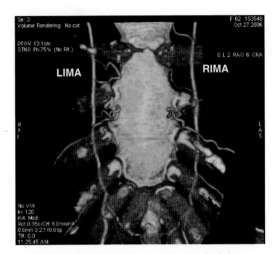

Figure 10.1 3D volume rendering showing the left internal mammary artery (LIMA) and the right internal mammary artery (RIMA) from the inside.

segments of the subclavian arteries) to the peripheral coronary arteries. A good knowledge of the various possible configurations and the operative report are the requisites for a successful mental and morphological reconstruction of every individual surgical procedure, which is the basis for the subsequent identification of occluded, failing or stenosed grafts.

Coronary artery bypass grafts can be venous or arterial vessels taken from the patient during the surgical procedure. The veins used most frequently for this purpose are the great saphenous veins (Figs. 10.5 and 10.6a,b). Commonly used arterial grafts are the left and right internal mammary arteries (Figs. 10.7, 10.8a,b, and 10.9), the radial arteries and, less commonly, the right gastroepiploic artery (Fig. 10.10). The internal mammary arteries can be utilized as *in situ* or "free" grafts: *in situ* means that their origin from the subclavian artery is preserved and the artery is surgically prepared (i.e., freed from its side branches)

Anatomy of the Heart by Multislice Computed Tomography. By Francesco Fulvio Faletra, Natesa G. Pandian and Siew Yen Ho. Published 2008 by Wiley-Blackwell Publishing, ISBN: 978-1-4051-8055-9.

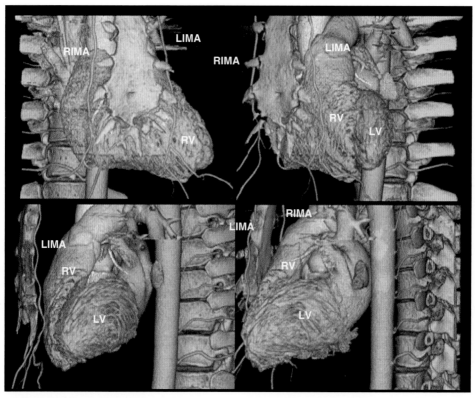

Figure 10.2 Electronic cast from different perspectives showing the left internal mammary artery (LIMA) and the right internal mammary artery (RIMA) and their relationships with the cast of right ventricular (RV) and left ventricular (LV) cavities.

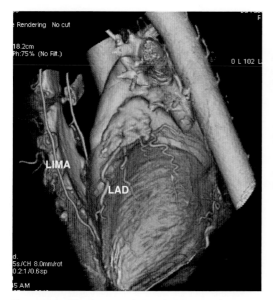

Figure 10.3 3D volume rendering showing the close relationship between the left internal mammary artery (LIMA) and the left anterior descending artery (LAD).

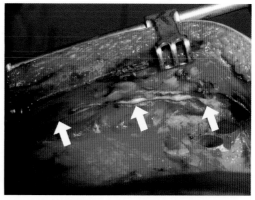

Figure 10.4 Image of the left internal mammary artery in the operating room.

and mobilized onto the heart for connection with the coronary artery that is to be bypassed (Figs. 10.7 and 10.8a,b). In this case, arterial blood flows from the aorta through the subclavian artery and the internal mammary artery into the bypassed coronary artery. A "free" graft means that the internal mammary artery is detached at its origin, transferred and interposed between another major arterial inflow vessel and the coronary artery.

Generally, coronary artery bypass grafts are connected proximally (i.e., centrally) to an arterial

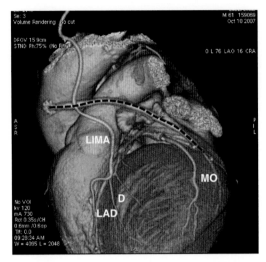

Figure 10.5   3D volume rendering showing a saphenous vein (broken line) used as a bypass graft connecting the aorta with the obtuse marginal branch (MO). The patient also has a left internal mammary artery (LIMA) that connects with the diagonal branch (D) and left descending artery (LAD).

vessel for inflow – this is called the "proximal anastomosis" (Figs. 10.11 and 10.12a,b). Most frequently, the proximal anastomosis is onto the ascending aorta as a termino-lateral anastomosis. Other anatomic sites for the proximal anastomosis can be the first few centimeters of the brachiocephalic trunk (accessible by median sternotomy) or, less frequently, the aortic arch or even the descending aorta and the left subclavian artery. There are also "non-anatomical" choices for the proximal anastomosis: bypass grafts themselves can serve as inflow for other bypass grafts. This results in the so-called Y- or T-configurations. Frequent examples are Y- or T-grafts taken off the left or right *in situ* internal mammary arteries. These grafts are usually arterial grafts. The Y- or T-anastomosis is intra-pericardial, that is on the more distal third of the "donating" graft. Vein grafts connected proximally to the ascending aorta can also serve as a "landing zone" for the proximal anastomosis of free arterial or other venous grafts (Fig. 10.13). There are many reasons for the confusing variability of the proximal anastomoses; for example, the relatively short anatomic length of a free arterial graft (i.e., the graft cannot reach the ascending aorta so it is connected to an internal mammary artery instead) or the surgeon's decision not to clamp the diseased ascending aorta for constructing a proximal anastomosis so

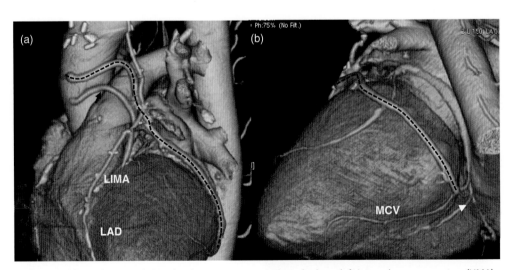

Figure 10.6   (a,b) 3D volume rendering showing a saphenous vein (broken line) used as bypass graft connecting the aorta (red arrow in (a)) with the right posterior descending artery (white arrow in (b)). The patient also has a left internal mammary artery (LIMA) connecting to the left descending artery (LAD) and a radial artery (black arrow) onto the intermediate branch (not seen in the image).

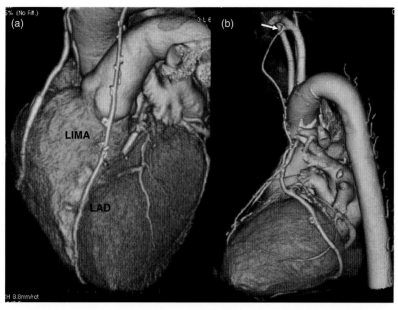

Figure 10.7   (a) 3D volume rendering showing the left internal mammary artery (LIMA) connecting with the left anterior descending artery (LAD). (b) The graft *in situ* (arrow); its origin from the subclavian artery is preserved.

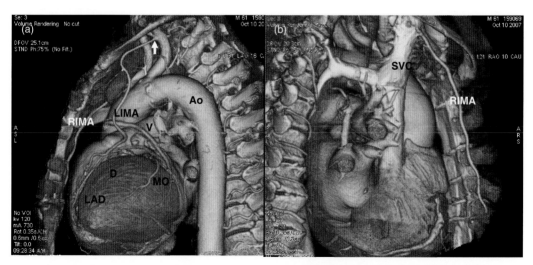

Figure 10.8   (a) Left anterior oblique view. 3D volume rendering showing the internal mammary artery (LIMA) originating from the subclavian artery (arrow) connecting with the first diagonal (D) and left anterior descending artery (LAD) and a venous bypass graft (V) connecting the aorta (Ao) with the marginal branch (MO). (b) Postero-lateral view showing the right internal mammary artery (RIMA). SVC = superior vena cava.

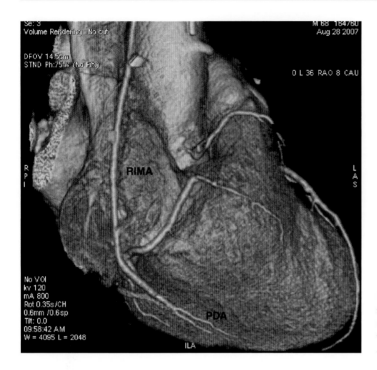

Figure 10.9   3D volume rendering showing the right internal mammary artery (RIMA) connecting with the right posterior descending artery (PDA).

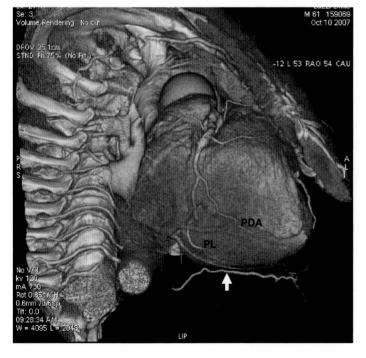

Figure 10.10   3D volume rendering. Lateral inferior view showing a segment of the gastroepiploic artery (arrow) and its proximity with the posterior descending artery (PDA) and postero-lateral branch (PL).

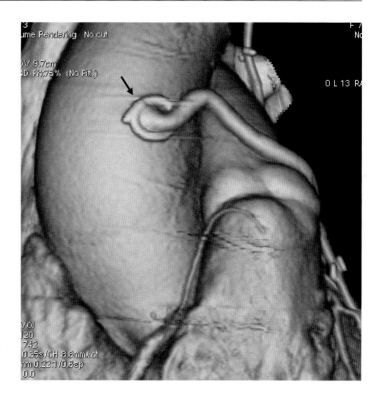

Figure 10.11   3D volume rendering showing the proximal anastomosis of venous graft.

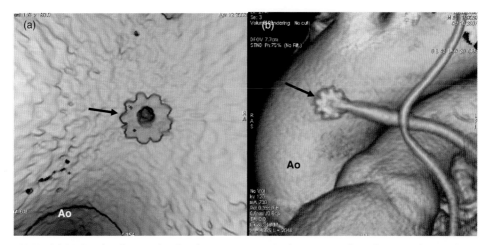

Figure 10.12   (a) 3D virtual endoscopy showing the proximal anastomosis (arrow) of venous graft as seen from the inside of the aorta. (b) 3D volume rendering; the same proximal anastomosis from the external antero-lateral perspective (arrow). Ao = aorta.

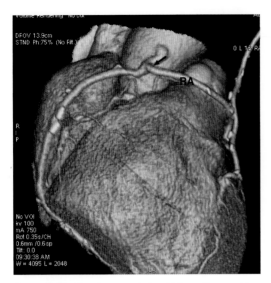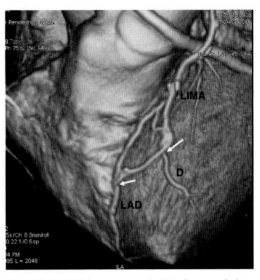

Figure 10.13   3D volume rendering. Vein graft connecting proximally to the ascending aorta serves as a "landing zone" for the proximal anastomosis of free radial artery (RA and arrow).

Figure 10.14   Distal anastomoses in 3D volume rendering of the left internal mammary artery (LIMA) on the diagonal branch (D) and on the left descending coronary artery (LDA).

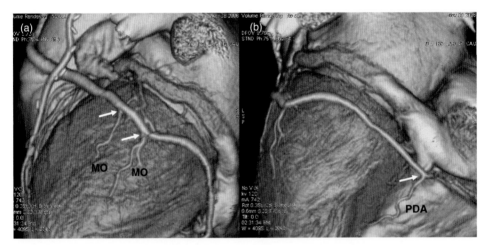

Figure 10.15   Distal anastomoses in 3D volume rendering. (a) A venous bypass graft with two latero-lateral anastomoses (arrows) on the marginal branches (MO).

(b) The termino-terminal anastomosis on the posterior descending artery (PDA).

as to reduce the risk of provoking cerebral atheromatous embolism.

All grafts are connected distally to one or more coronary arteries, the so-called "distal anastomosis." When grafts are connected with more coronary arteries the graft is called a "sequential" or "jump" graft and there are one or more latero-lateral anastomoses (along the epicardial course of the graft) and one termino-lateral anastomosis (the most distal site) (Figs. 10.14 and 10.15).

Index